Healing with Chinese Herbs

by
Lesley Gunsaulus Tierra, L. Ac., Dip. Ac.

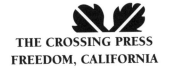

THE CROSSING PRESS
FREEDOM, CALIFORNIA

For information on bulk purchases or group discounts for this and other Crossing Press titles, please contact our Special Sales Manager at 800-777-1048.

ISBN 0-89594-829-X

*To the Divine Mother
and all healing plants*

*I give many thanks to my husband, Michael Tierra,
an avid teacher and inspiring practitioner,
whose vision and love first introduced me to the teachings
and the way of life of Traditional Chinese Medicine.*

Contents

Introduction

Traditional Chinese herbal medicine has been practiced for over 4000 years. It employs a highly developed theoretical system, which determines the appropriate application of herbs. Traditional Chinese Medicine (also known as "TCM") teaches that the causes of disease are various, and that symptoms differ according to the individual. As a result, TCM treats the causes of disease and not the diseases themselves. Thus, even seemingly incurable conditions can be healed. The theoretical foundation of TCM takes the various causes of disease into account; it helps herbalists to recognize the various patterns the causes of disease can form, and trains them to recognize the specific qualities and uses of each herb.

For example, rather than making a headache the main treatment focus, we look at the person to see what is occurring in the body to cause the headache. Causes may include liver congestion, stomach upset, tension, or bodily weakness. These causes vary according to the individual's body and existing health imbalances. The herbal treatment also varies: dandelion relieves headaches caused by liver congestion, chrysanthemum alleviates headaches due to stomach upset, oyster shell can ease tension headaches, and cinnamon can eliminate headaches resulting from bodily weakness. Each of the above-named herbs is different, and each of them regulates a headache in its own way. This approach differs significantly from giving a single medication (such as willow bark) for all types of headaches.

TCM developed through the empirical method, which determines truth or knowledge through observation, experience, and experiments. Knowledge of the organ systems and their influences, the causes of disease, methods of herb application, and the healing effects of herbs were developed through thousands of years of observation, experience, and experiments.

Today, science is based on systematic experiments; these experiments, in turn, are focused on measuring, quantifying, and separating the whole into parts. While these methods have led to the technical revolution, they have also become exclusive. Within this framework, the knowledge we gain through experience is no longer sufficient; our senses have been replaced by laboratory experiments. Unfortunately, Western scientific methodology has eliminated the application of empirical evidence and eradicated thousands of years of multicultural experience; this is a true loss to modern society.

As a result, Traditional Chinese Medicine has increasingly found its way into Western cultures. It provides specific answers and cures not found in Western medicine. Additionally, herbalism does not create the side effects or sensitivities caused by Western medication. In short, this system of ancient medicine has much to offer the West.

In China, Western and Chinese medicines are used hand in hand, drawing on one another's advantages. Chinese hospitals employ both Western and Chinese practitioners. Acupuncture anesthesia and herbal recovery enhance surgery, the crowning glory of Western medicine. Other healing centers use acupuncture, herbalism, and other healing modalities in place of surgery.

Traditional Chinese Medicine asserts that daily participation in the martial-arts movements of *Qi Gong* and *Tai Chi Chuan*, the use of medicinal herbs, and the adoption of appropriate lifestyle habits—including a healthful diet, adequate physical activity, sexual expression, and moderate bedtime hours—all prevent disease. In Chinese life, herbs are used on an almost daily basis. Families consume herbal soup weekly, or even daily, which aids their adjustment to seasonal and environmental changes. This preventative measure keeps the entire family well.

I have studied, practiced, and included TCM in my life for at least 16 years. Over and over I have seen, for myself and thousands of patients, that its theories and practices bring answers, healing, and a richness of life not found in Western society. The use of herbs—in and of itself—can be helpful, but its effectiveness is greatly enhanced when combined with appropriate diet and lifestyle habits. Many patients ask me, "Why didn't anyone tell me these things? Why did I have to find out the hard way?" My response is this: Although these ancient truths are no longer a part of our society, we can empower ourselves with the wisdom of our ancestors, and learn from them now.

Accordingly, I wrote this guide as a reference to the theoretical foundation and application of Traditional Chinese Medicine. It is intended as both an educational and practical guide to the daily use of herbs. The culinary use of herbs, patent herbal medicines, descriptions of individual herbs, and remedies for common ailments are strongly emphasized. To delve deeper into TCM, readers should review the "Recommended Reading and Sources" guide, on page 188.

Learning about Chinese herbs can be simple. It can also be a joyous, life-long, complex pursuit. I am sure you will feel enriched and rewarded, however you wish to embrace Chinese herbalism.

Questions About Chinese Herbal Medicine

Q. *Why use Chinese herbs?*
Chinese herbs have been used in the healing process for approximately 4000 years. There are many external and internal applications for various herbs but a particular category of Chinese herbs, called tonics, has proven uniquely effective. Tonic herbs are divided into four subcategories: tonics for energy (*qi*); blood; the warming activating functions of the body (*yang*); and the cooling, moistening functions of the body (*yin*).

Q. *What are the differences between Chinese and Western herbalism?*
Understanding and use of traditional Chinese herbs are based on a particular theoretical foundation, as follows: first, an individual's constitution is determined; then, the energy of the disease is evaluated; and finally, herbs are chosen that match the energy of both the person and the disease.

At one time, Hippocrates' Greek humour system was the theoretical basis for traditional Western herbalism. In this system, people and their diseases were evaluated according to their energies, and the appropriate herbs were chosen on the basis of such energy. The seventeenth and eighteenth centuries, however, saw the advent of materialistic thinking and Cartesian principles; as a result, the West formed a mechanistic view of nature and the theoretical system of humours was lost.

Modern medicine and Western herbalism view and treat disease separately from the person who experiences it. In the treatment of disease, herbs are applied solely according to their therapeutic properties and chemical constituents. Disease is separated from the individual, and a plant is broken down into components, rather than using the whole. In Western herbal treatment, the disease is identified and given common treatment. Everyone who receives the same diagnosis gets the same cure.

In Chinese herbalism, people who appear to have the same illness are treated with different herbs and formulas, according to the presence of hot, cold, dry, damp, or other energies. These energies cause specific types of illness in each person.

Q. Are Chinese herbs safe to take internally?
Herbs are generally mild, like special foods. With few exceptions, they lack the concentration of active biochemical ingredients. Herbs possess constituents that counterbalance and enhance one another's effectiveness. An herbal formula, or combination, acts in synergy: it buffers the strong effects of individual herbs while it enhances each of their functions and purposes. When herbs interact with the innate functional processes of the body, they regulate chemical physiological imbalances; for the most part, they do not cause severe, long-term, adverse reactions. Herbs can be powerful, however, and should be used with knowledge.

Q. Can I use Chinese herbs while taking my medication?
Almost all Chinese herbs can be taken with Western medications. However, it may take longer for the herbs to be effective. If you are taking medication to treat a serious condition, consult a Chinese herbal practitioner before starting a complex herbal formula. In general, it is safe to take simple, one- to two-herb formulas in conjunction with Western medication.

Q. Where do Chinese herbs come from?
Most Chinese herbs, liquid extracts, and pills come from Taiwan or mainland China. However, an increasing number of Chinese herbs are currrently grown in the United States.

Q. Where do I find Chinese herbs?
Chinese herbs are readily available in the Chinatowns of major cities, including San Francisco, New York, and St. Louis. They can also be purchased,

through mail order, in pill, tablet, bulk-herb, powdered extract and formula form. Several herbal sources are listed in the "Recommended Reading and Sources" guide on page 188.

Q. Are Chinese herbs sprayed?

Many Chinese herbs are sprayed with sulfites to fulfill the United States' importation requirements. However, it is now often possible to find unsprayed herbs. Some of these herbs are available on the market from Chinese herbal companies. (Several of these companies are listed in the "Recommended Reading and Sources" section, on page 188.) Further, there has been no noted reaction to sprayed Chinese herbs. Their effectiveness far outweighs the possible dangers of fumigation, and benefits even the most sensitive bodies. I have seen several people with severe environmental and food allergies profit from sprayed Chinese herbs, without experiencing side effects. I have also seen individuals suffering from serious ailments, such as walking pneumonia, respond to sprayed herbs with no ill results.

Q. What is the safest, most effective form of Chinese herbs?

Tea is the most effective form in which to take Chinese herbs, since it is highly assimilable by the body. However, many people find its taste strange or unpleasant. Liquid extracts, powdered extracts, pills, and tablets are also effective and readily available.

Q. How do I determine which herbs to use?

Determination of herb usage involves three elements. An individual's energy and the energy of the disease must first be evaluated. Appropriate herbal energies are then chosen in accordance with these elements. Information on this evaluation process is given in the chapter entitled "Determining Which Herbs to Use," beginning on page 18.

Q. What are Chinese tonic herbs?

Tonic herbs strengthen and enhance the functioning of a certain part of the body. Chinese tonic herbs are unique to Western herbalism, because few Western herbs that fulfill these functions have been identified. Chinese tonics are categorized as follows: those herbs that strengthen and build blood; energy (*qi*); the activating and warming functions of the body (*yang*); and the cooling and moistening functions of the body (*yin*).

Q. How are herbs classified by energy?

Almost all traditional herbal systems classify herbs and foods according to their heating or cooling energies, flavors, directions, the organs they specifically influence, and their other properties. The cooling energy lowers metabolism and clears heat, such as fevers. The warming energy increases metabolism, warms the body, and activates physiological processes. Herbs with pungent and sweet flavors have a warming energy, while those with sour, salty, or bitter flavors have cooling energies.

An herb's direction refers to its ability to influence the exterior or interior of the body: to move energy, blood, and fluids (such as expectorants) upwards, or downwards (in the case of diuretics or laxatives). Additionally, herbs generally influence specific organs in the body and aid their functions. Some herbs (such as Siberian ginseng) enable the body to withstand stress, or (in the case of astragalus, reishi mushrooms, and Korean ginseng) enhance immune potential.

Q. Why are most traditional herbs taken in complex formulas?

Generally, the sum effect of all the herbs in a formula is greater than the potency of herbs taken individually. In a formula, the various properties of the herbs interact with each other to enhance and strengthen their therapeutic effects. Thus, complex formulas are generally more effective than single herbs. If a health condition is simple, one herb may be enough. If the condition is complex, herbs taken together are more effective.

Chinese Herbal Fundamentals

The theoretical foundation of Chinese medicine is based upon the concepts of *yin*, *yang*, *qi*, blood, fluids, Essence, and *Shen*. All treatment through food and herbs is founded upon these ideas. Although these concepts may seem strange to the Western mind, they can be easily grasped. Repeated reading and application of these principles make them easier to understand, and, in time, they can become part of one's life view.

Yin and Yang

Yin is fluidic, cooling, and equated with hypo-metabolic qualities and conditions. Physiologically, it represents the body's substance, including blood and all other fluids in the body. *Yin* nourishes, nurtures, and moistens all aspects of the body, including organs and tissues.

Yang represents the body's capacity to generate and maintain warmth. It can be equated with hyper-metabolic qualities that affect all organic processes, including warmth, libido, appetite, digestion, and assimilation. Its normal manifestation is comparable to our concept of zest for life.

The ancient Chinese applied the concepts of *yin* and *yang* to all aspects of natural phenomena. *Yin* represents the earth, moon, and the material, while *yang* represents heaven, the sun, and the immaterial. Their qualities are as follows:

Qualities of Yin and Yang		
	Yin	**Yang**
action	rest	activity
tendency	condense, contract	develop, expand
color	dark	bright
temperature	cold	hot
weight	heavy	light
catalyst	water	fire
light	dark	light
work	psychological	physical
attitude	introvert	extrovert
energy	receptive	aggressive
nerves	parasympathetic	sympathetic
tastes	sour, bitter, salty	spicy, sweet
season	winter	summer

Qi

Qi is another word for the energy, vital force, or life force that pervades all of life. In the body it is given different names according to its various functions and forms. *Qi* warms the body and the digestion; it acts as the metabolic fire for food and fluids; it circulates blood and fluids, spreading them throughout the organs, cells, muscles, tissues, and limbs of the body; it holds the organs in their proper places and retains blood in the vessels; it transforms one substance into another; lastly, it protects the body from the "invasion" of colds, flu, fevers, and other "bugs," as we call them in the West.

Qi has an intimate relationship with blood. In fact, *qi* and blood are seen as interrelated and interdependent. This life force circulates blood, helps to create blood from food and drink, and holds blood in the vessels. On the other hand, blood nourishes *qi*.

Qi can be congested or weak. Symptoms of weak or deficient *qi* are low vitality; lethargy; shortness of breath; slow metabolism; slow recovery from frequent colds and flu; a low, soft voice; spontaneous sweating; frequent urination; and palpitations. Examples of herbs that strengthen *qi* include astragalus, Chinese wild yam, codonopsis, ginseng, and jujube dates.

Blood

Traditional Chinese Medicine conceives of blood as similar, though broader in definition, to the blood in our vessels. It is a very dense and material form of *qi*. Blood warms the body; moistens tissues, muscles, skin, and hair; and, most importantly, nourishes the cells and organs. Blood has an interdependent relationship with *qi*; it depends on the circulating function of *qi* to spread it throughout all parts of the body. Blood, however, nourishes and supports *qi*, giving it life and movement.

Blood can be congested, weak, or contain excessive heat (such as toxins). Symptoms of weak or deficient blood include dizziness; amenorrhea (or scanty menses); an emaciated body; the appearance of spots in the visual field; impaired vision; numb arms or legs; dry skin, hair, or eyes; a lusterless, pale face and lips; fatigue; and poor memory. *Dong quai*, lycii berries, longan berries, cooked rehmannia, and white peony all strengthen the blood.

Fluids

Fluids are also known as body fluids. They encompass all fluids in the body other than blood, including cerebrospinal fluid; interstitial fluid; intracellular fluid; saliva; sweat; urine; tears; and all bodily excretions and secretions, such as mucus, phlegm, and lymph fluid. Fluids nurture, moisten, and lubricate all parts of the body. They are divided into pure and impure parts. The pure parts are recycled in the body, while the impure ones are discharged as urine.

Fluids can be deficient, excessive, or congested. A deficiency of fluids, or dryness, results in the following symptoms: dry, rough, chapped, or cracked skin; dry throat, nose, mouth, or lips; dry coughing with minimal phlegm; dry stools; dehydration; and unusual thirst. *Yin* tonics generally moisten and cool while they clear heat. Chinese asparagus, dendrobium, lily bulb, and ophio-pogon are examples of moistening herbs.

An excess of fluid results in copious bodily excretions, such as lung phlegm or vaginal discharge; loose stools; a feeling of heaviness in any part of the body; oozing skin eruptions; edema; abdominal distension; chest fullness; nausea; and sore, heavy, or stiff joints. Atractylodis, cardamom, coix, fritillar-ia, hoelen, and platycodon dry up excessive dampness in the body.

Essence

Essence (also called *jing*) is the basis of reproduction, development, growth, sexual power, conception, pregnancy, and decay in the body. It includes semen and the reproductive capacity of the body. Essence also forms our basic consti-tutional strength and vitality. In its broadest and most comprehensive sense, "Essence" refers to the overall hormonal strength that regulates normal growth, metabolism, and sexuality. Although it is not a fluid, Essence is fluid-like and considered a part of *yin*. It is stored in the kidney-adrenals.

Symptoms of Essence-deficiency include premature aging, senility, bad or loose teeth, poor memory or concentration, brittle or soft bones, weakness of knees and legs, loss of hair, premature graying of hair, low libido or impotence, three or more miscarriages, infertility, and wasting of flesh. Various *yin*, *yang*, blood, and *qi* tonics—such as cuscuta, epemedium, *he shou wu*, and polygo-nati—nourish Essence.

Shen

Shen encompasses both Mind and Spirit. It reflects the entire physical, emo-tional, mental, and spiritual health of the body. The principle of *Shen* involves the capacity to think and act coherently, the force of human personality, and joy in living. It also includes the spiritual aspects of all the organs. The pres-ence of *Shen* is distinguished by sparkling eyes, an overall vivaciousness, and the will to live. *Shen* is housed in the heart.

Physical *Shen*-deficiency does not exist, since *Shen* disharmony is spiritu-al. However, since this principle is connected with the heart, insufficient *qi* or blood of the heart could cause a weakness of *Shen*. Symptoms of this condi-tion include dull eyes, dislike of talking, disinterest in life, muddled thinking, forgetfulness, insomnia, lack of vitality, depression, unhappiness, confused speech, or excessive dreaming. An extreme *Shen* imbalance can result in irrational behavior, incoherent speech, unconsciousness, hysteria, delirium, inappropriate responses, and violent madness.

Biota seeds, longan berries, polygala, and zizyphus seeds—which also feed the heart—help nourish the *Shen*. True remedies for *Shen* weakness include addressing spiritual issues through life counseling; prayer, affirmation, and meditation practices; increased play; career changes; taking a holiday; and other actions that nourish the Spirit and heart.

Determining Which Herbs to Use

Traditional Chinese Medicine uses a system called the Eight Principles to identify the location, energy, and severity of an illness. Once this system is applied, it is easy to determine the appropriate herbs for treatment. The structure of this system indicates that TCM does not treat disease itself; rather, it treats the causes of illness. Definitions of the Eight Principles are as follows:

THE EIGHT PRINCIPLES	
external	surface of the body: colds, flu, fevers, skin eruptions, sore throats, headaches
internal	interior of the body: conditions affecting the *qi*, blood, fluids, and internal organs
excess	congestion of *qi*, blood, fluids, or excessive cold or heat in the body
deficiency	lack of *qi*, blood, fluids, *yin*, or *yang* in the body
hot	overactive metabolism
cold	low metabolism
yang	body's capacity to generate and maintain warmth; hypermetabolic
yin	fluidic, cooling body's substance; hypometabolic

External and Internal

External and internal refer to the location of an illness in the body. In general, internal conditions tend to be chronic, while external conditions are acute.

External conditions are located on the surface of the body and affect the upper respiratory passages, including the nasal passages, mouth, throat, bronchioles, and lungs; the skin; and hair. These conditions include the acute manifestations of colds, flu, fevers, skin eruptions, acute arthritic conditions, and injuries. To alleviate external diseases, induce sweating. Chrysanthemum, cinnamon twigs, ginger, honeysuckle, and mint effectively treat such external conditions.

Internal syndromes affect the *qi*, blood, body fluids, and internal organs. The symptomology of such conditions can include constipation, gastritis, ulcers, urinary infections, low energy, weakness, diabetes, hypoglycemia, cancer, epilepsy, gynecological conditions, infertility, impotence, and heart disease. TCM diagnosis of these conditions determines the appropriate herbs to use in their treatment. Herbs are selected according to their heating or cooling energies; which organs they enter; and whether they eliminate, strengthen, or move *qi*, blood, and fluids.

It is possible to simultaneously experience an acute and an internal condition. For example, an individual may suffer from a cold or flu while dealing with poor digestion or menstrual irregularity. In such cases, the acute external condition must be treated before the internal condition.

Excess and Deficiency

Excess and deficiency describe a person's strength and weakness in relation to their illness.

Excess is a congested state of *qi*, blood, fluids, cold, or food. Its symptoms include obesity, constipation, hypertension, severe infections, purulent discharges, and edema. Herbs that dry dampness, remove congestion, detoxify, and eliminate and clear heat, and herbs that circulate *qi*, blood, and fluids are used to treat excessive conditions. Generally, treatment of excess patterns is easier than treatment of deficient conditions, because the elimination of substances is quicker and simpler than building the *qi*, blood, *yin*, or *yang* of the body.

Deficiency is a lack of *qi*, blood, *yin*, *yang*, or Essence. Individuals with deficient conditions generally have weakened immune systems, and are hypersensitive to stress, climate, and foods. Typically, recovery from deficient conditions takes longer than recovery from excessive conditions. Manifestations of a deficient condition may include fatigue, weakness, weak digestion, a low presence of hydrochloric acid, hypothyroidism, hypoadrenalism, anemia, and wasting diseases such as tuberculosis and AIDS. Tonic herbs strengthen the *qi*, blood, *yin*, *yang*, or Essence.

Hot and Cold

Hot and cold refer to the body's innate metabolism.

Heat represents hypermetabolism, and is a part of *yang*. Symptoms may include sensations of heat; inflammation; a ruddy complexion; reddened eyes; restlessness; an aggressive manner; a loud voice; constipation; thirst; scanty, dark-yellow or red urine; a desire for cold; an aversion to heat; the discharge of yellow mucus, stools, or vaginal secretions; the discharge of dark-yellow or red-tinged urine; bloody discharges; burning digestion; infections; inflammations; internal or external dryness; hemorrhaging; irritability; profuse sweating; a strong appetite; fever; and hyperconditions, such as hypertension.

Coldness is a part of *yin*, and represents a lowered metabolism. Symptoms include sensations of cold; a pale complexion; lethargy; weak digestion; low immunity; an aversion to cold and a desire for warmth; severe chills; lack of thirst or sweating; slowness in movement, speech, or body functions; diarrhea or loose stools; excessive sleep; poor circulation; low blood pressure; poor appetite; expectoration of clear-to-white mucus; discharge of clear-to-white vaginal fluids; joint pain; frequent, copious, and clear urination; nighttime urination; frigidity; impotence; infertility; anemia; and all hypoconditions, such as hypoadrenalism, hypoglycemia, and hypothyroidism.

Yin and Yang

Yin and *yang* are a summation of the preceding conditions.

Yang represents a composite of external, excessive, or hot symptoms or conditions. Other *yang* conditions include hypertension, hyperadrenalism, and hyperthyroidism; and overbearing, aggressive behavior.

Yin encompasses a composite of the symptoms or conditions that are internal, deficient, or cold. Other *yin* conditions include endocrine imbalances associated with hypothyroidism, hypoadrenalism, and hypoglycemia; a pale complexion; fluid retention; timidity; and the presence of a soft voice.

There are four possible imbalances of *yang* and *yin*: *yang*-excess, *yang*-deficiency, *yin*-excess, and *yin*-deficiency.

Yang-excess: This condition is identical to excess heat. It is accompanied by symptoms of high fever, restlessness, a red complexion, a loud voice, aggressive actions, emission of strong odors, release of yellow discharges, rapid pulse, and hypertension. Herbs such as chrysanthemum flowers, honeysuckle, and rhubarb root—which detoxify, clear heat, and promote bowel movements—are most useful in the treatment of this condition.

Yang-deficiency: A *yang*-deficiency manifests itself in symptoms of lethargy, a feeling of coldness, edema, poor digestion, lower-back pain, constipation caused by weak peristaltic motion, and lack of libido. In *yang*-deficiency, the heat and activity necessary to perform adequate body functions are absent. Herbs such as ginger, cinnamon, and *yang* tonics (like cuscuta, psoralea, and eucommia) that treat coldness and warm the body should be used to counteract this condition.

Yin-excess: *Yin*-excess is a condition of internal dampness, which includes symptoms of excessive fluid retention; lethargy; a plump or generally swollen appearance; and overall signs of dampness, including feelings of heaviness, lung or sinus phlegm, excessive vaginal discharge, mucus in the stools, and edema. Individuals with a *yin*-excess, however, may have adequate energy. In such cases, spicy, warm-natured herbs such as cinnamon and ginger, and diuretics such as hoelen help promote the elimination of excess water.

Yin-deficiency: This condition is one of deficient heat. It results in emaciation and weakness, and is accompanied (surprisingly) by heat symptoms. In *yin*-deficiency, heat symptoms occur in the absence of cooling, moistening fluids (*yin*). This condition is termed "false heat." A person with *yin*-deficiency may be emaciated; exhibit nervous energy; talk quickly but tire rapidly; sleep poorly; and lack stamina and resistance. Other symptoms include night sweats; insomnia; a burning sensation in the palms, soles, or chest; a malar flush; afternoon fevers; nervous exhaustion; a dry throat; dry eyes; blurred vision; dizziness; and nervous tension. *Yin*-tonifying herbs include Chinese asparagus and ophiopogon.

An excess of *yang* and a deficiency of *yin* are both associated with excessive heat, irritability, and other *yang* symptoms. In each case, however, these symptoms arise from entirely different imbalances; as such, these syndromes are not identical. *Yang*-excess is accompanied by true heat signs. *Yin*-deficiency manifests itself in an underlying weakness accompanied by superficial heat signs, such as flushed cheeks; night sweats; and burning sensations in the palms, soles, or chest.

Similarly, a *yang*-deficiency exhibits symptoms similar to those of a *yin*-excess. These conditions are not identical, however, because they originate (respectively) from points of deficiency or excess. In a *yang*-deficiency, where heat and activity are not sufficient to provide energy or transform fluids, symptoms include a feeling of coldness and organ hypofunction. *Yin*-excess, on the other hand, results in significant bodily dampness, including copious discharges and a full, rounded body.

Combination of Patterns

There can be combinations of more than one imbalance. Some examples of these are:

External-Excess-Heat: This condition has symptoms of skin eruptions; rashes; boils; eczema; strong body odor; restless sleep; anxiety; yellowish mucus, which may be red-tinged with blood; loud and strong breathing; scanty, dark-colored urination; and possible constipation or diarrhea. If an individual experiencing this condition has a fever, it tends to be high. Use cooling herbs that treat the exterior, herbs that clear heat, antispasmodics, diuretics, nervines, expectorants, purgatives, or astringents.

External-Excess-Cold: Characteristics of this condition often include a feeling of coldness; general stiffness; slow movement; lowered immunity; aversion to cold, wind, and damp; lack of sweating; low-grade fever and chills; a pale, puffy complexion; drowsiness; clear or cloudy-white mucus; strong and labored breathing; light-colored, frequent urination; and normal-to-loose stools. To treat this condition, use herbs with a warming energy (including diuretics, expectorants, aromatic stomachics, and astringents), which treat the exterior.

External-Deficient-Heat: An individual with this condition may be frail, thin, restless, anxious; experience mood changes, lowered immunity, aversion to heat and wind, restless sleep, thirst, spontaneous perspiration, night sweats, a low-grade fever, acute or chronic recurring sore throats. This is a *yin*-deficient condition, which should be treated with *yin* tonic herbs.

External-Deficient-Cold: This condition's symptoms include a feeling of coldness; frailness; anemia; a pale complexion; thinness; insecurity; sadness or depression; low immunity; expectoration of clear or whitish mucus; lack of thirst; acute conditions that tend to arise quickly and are accompanied by a mild fever and stronger chills; shallow breath; explusion of loose stools; and a tendency to sleep frequently. To prevent this condition, use warming herbs that treat the exterior, warm the body, and circulate energy.

Internal-Deficient-Cold: Symptoms of this deficiency include coldness; low energy characterized by the symptoms of hypothyroidism or hypoadrenalism; timidity; a pale complexion; anemia; lack of thirst; recurring colds and flu; sleepiness; thin, clear mucus discharges; pale and wet lips; shallow or weak breathing; low libido; joint and lower-back pain; pale, scant, late, or irregular menstruation; frequent and copious urination, possibly at night; and loose stools. This is a *yang* deficiency, which is treated with *qi* and *yang* tonics and warming diuretics.

Internal-Excess-Cold: The symptoms of this excess may include a feeling of coldness; cold extremities; pale complexion; flaccidity; severe edema; slow movement; melancholia; alternating moods; aversion to cold and dampness; poor digestion, with gas and bloating; expectoration of clear or white mucus; allergies; a short menstrual cycle; slow menstrual bleeding with possible dull pain; the presence of light-colored, copious urination, possibly at night; and the expulsion of loose stools. This is an excess of *yin*, and should be treated with warming stimulants, aromatic stomachics, diuretics, and *yang* and *qi* tonics.

Internal-Excess-Heat: Individuals with this condition may exhibit bloody stools, urine, vomit, or expectorations; vomiting; strong body odors; aversion to heat; irritability and aggressive temperament; energetic activity, and a tendency towards insomnia; loud, commanding speech; strong appetite; excessive thirst; heavy, coarse breathing; infections and inflammations; strong sexual drive; yellow- or red-colored eyes; dry, cracked lips; heavy menses (generally early and long in duration); emission of dark-colored urination; expulsion of hard stools; constipation; or hot, yellow diarrhea. This is *yang* excess. It is treated with cooling herbs: purgative herbs or herbs that clear heat and dampness.

Internal-Deficient-Heat: Symptoms include lowered immunity; thinness; restlessness; lack of stamina; thirst; night sweats; restless sleep; weak digestion; low-grade infections; burning sensations in palms of the hands, soles of the feet, or chest; thin, yellowish urination, recurring bladder infections, and constipation; and light, short, irregular, painful menstruation. This is a *yin* deficiency; it should be treated with *yin* tonics, herbs that clear heat and cool blood, nervines, sedatives, and calmatives.

Herbal Properties

The various aspects of herbs give each herb its unique personality and use, and they determine conditions in which the herb is effective or ineffective. These aspects are listed below:

- heating or cooling energy
- the five tastes
- the four directions
- affected organs and meridians

Heating or Cooling Energy

An herb's energy is hot, warm, neutral, cool, or cold. Hot and cold herbs are very rare; the use of warming or cooling energies is more common. Neutral energy is balanced; it neither warms nor cools the body.

An herb's heating energy warms the body, stimulates circulation and metabolism, and gives energy. An herb's cooling energy cools the body, slows metabolism, and clears heat. Herbs with a heating or warming energy are used when symptoms such as coldness and lowered metabolism appear, and herbs with a cooling energy are employed when symptoms of heat and hypermetabolism are present.

The Five Tastes

An herb's taste helps determine its heating or cooling energy. Taste gives various qualities and effects to a particular herb, all of which indicate the use of the herb. In the West, there are four recognizable tastes. In the Orient, there are five tastes: sweet, bitter, pungent, salty, and sour.

The energy and taste of various herbs are assimilated into the body and nourish different organs. The lungs and large intestine absorb pungent tastes; kidneys and urinary bladder absorb salty tastes; liver and gallbladder absorb sour tastes; heart and small intestine absorb bitter tastes; and spleen and stomach absorb sweet tastes.

These five tastes have a therapeutic use. Specific organs are strengthened by a small amount of the corresponding taste, but weakened by an excess of the same taste. A small exposure to sweet taste strengthens the spleen and stomach, and the body's digestive capacity. However, an excess of sweet taste (over time) weakens the body's ability to digest and assimilate.

Pungent: The pungent taste, also called "acrid" or "spicy," generally has a warm-to-hot energy. It stimulates the circulation of blood; energy; lymphatic fluid; other fluids and secretions, such as sweat, saliva, and tears; and nerve energy. The pungent taste counteracts poor digestion and circulation, coldness, and mucus production. It moves energy from the inside to the outside of the body by opening pores and facilitating sweat. This taste is especially useful in counteracting surface ailments such as colds, flu, and mucus congestion. The spicy taste has a direct effect on the lungs and large intestine.

Since pungent herbs disperse energy and blood—especially to the surface of the body, where it often leaves through sweat—they can (in excess) exhaust energy reserves; cause fingernails and toenails to wither; and tighten the tendons, which decreases flexibility. As such, they should be used only as needed. Ginger, and black and red peppers are all herbs with the pungent taste.

Salty: The energy of the salty taste is cold, and it stabilizes and regulates fluid balance. It also has a softening effect, and is beneficial in treating hardened lymph nodes, tight muscles, constipation, hard lumps, masses, and cysts. The salty taste directly affects the kidneys, adrenals, and bladder. An excessive craving for salt may indicate impending adrenal exhaustion.

In excess, salt can cause water retention and high blood pressure. However, herbs that are high in mineral salts do not generate excess salt. Seaweeds, such as kelp, have a salty taste.

Sour: The sour taste is cooling, drying, astringent, and refreshing; it dries up mucus and tightens and tones tissues and muscles. Sour taste helps to stop bodily discharges such as excessive perspiration, diarrhea, seminal emission, spermatorrhea (frequent, involuntary loss of sperm without orgasm), frequent urination, copious mucus, and bleeding. It also stimulates digestion and metabolism. Through its stimulation of bile, the sour taste aids in the breakdown of fats and facilitates their absorption. The sour taste drains and expels excess in the liver and gallbladder.

In excess, however, the sour taste can actually harm digestion—it may coat the mucous linings of the stomach and intestines, causing poor digestion and absorption. The sour taste can also toughen the flesh. Herbs with the sour taste include schisandra and orange peel.

Bitter: This taste is cooling, drying, detoxifying, and anti-inflammatory. Bitter taste eliminates bodily dampness and secretions such as diarrhea, leukorrhea, and skin abscesses. It stimulates the secretion of bile, which in turn sparks digestive fires and stimulates normal bowel elimination. Bitter substances help protect the body against parasites and clears the blood of cholesterol. As such, the bitter taste strengthens the heart and small intestine, and cleanses the blood. Sweet cravings can be alleviated by ingesting the bitter taste.

Bitter subtances, in excess, can dry and eliminate to a detrimental extent. They may also cause the skin to wither and body hair to fall out. Bitter herbs include gentian, rhubarb, and apricot seed.

Sweet: The sweet taste is warming, tonifying, and harmonizing. Sweet-tasting herbs strengthen weak individuals with a lack of energy and blood; this is why people with low energy are drawn to sweets. However, these individuals generally choose simple sweets, such as sugary snacks. Ultimately, simple sweets *deplete* energy, by causing blood sugar to rise and drop sharply. Complex carbohydrates, protein, and sweet-tasting herbs strengthen the body and give it energy.

Excessive ingestion of the sweet taste can lead to congestion and lethargy, and may sedate the digestive fires. It may also cause aching bones and joints and hair loss. Ginseng, red dates, and cinnamon are sweet-tasting herbs.

The Four Directions

Each herb has a tendency to move in one of four directions within the body—rising or upward, sinking or downward, floating or outward, and descending or inward.

Rising or upward: Stimulating herbs have a rising energy, which helps remove obstructions and promotes circulation. Herbs with this energy include motherwort and black pepper.

Sinking or downward: The sinking energy causes urinary or intestinal elimination, activates menses, and lowers fevers. *Dang gui* and alisma have the sinking, or downward, energy.

Floating or outward: The floating energy disperses colds and flu to the outside of the body, and eliminates toxins through the pores of the skin. Herbs with volatile oils, such as fresh ginger and peppermint, have a floating energy.

Descending or inward: The descending energy strengthens the inner organs and enhances their functions. Herbs with descending, or inward, energy include ginseng and rehmannia.

An herb's preparation influences its directional energy. Herbal extracts combined with wine or alcohol have a rising tendency, since alcohol has a rising energy. Mixed with ginger juice, an herb generally moves to the body's extremities, because ginger is spicy and tends to disperse. Herbs taken in vinegar sink downward within the body, since vinegar's energy is heavy.

When herbs with a spicy, rising energy are combined with various other herbs, the resulting formula can—by ascending—treat the upper part of the body. The same principle (in reverse) applies when herbs with downward-moving energies are added to other herbs.

The energy of an herb and the energy of the disease it treats should be similar in direction. A superficial disease located in the upper part of the lungs, for example, should be treated with rising and floating herbs that cause sweating and mucus expectoration. Sinking herbs with laxative or diuretic properties are used in the treatment of intestinal or urinary-tract disease. Internal weakness (accompanied by poor digestion, lowered appetite, bloating, and gas) can be successfully treated with inward-moving, strengthening herbs.

Affected Organs and Meridians

Herbs are also defined by the particular effect they have on one or more organs. Chinese and Western views of physiology differ greatly. Traditional Chinese Medicine describes organs in terms of their energetic, rather than physical, functions: organs are understood through an observation of dynamic, interrelated processes that occur at every level and within every cell of the body, rather than through definitions of discrete, local, and specialized functions. Each internal organ is connected to numerous channels and collaterals, called meridians, which supply the organ with sustaining energy and nourishment. This theory of organs is called *Zang Fu*.

Organs are divided into two types: solid organs (*Zang*), which transform, and the hollow organs (*Fu*), which store. Solid organs are vital and considered *yin*; the hollow organs are functional and considered *yang*. *Yin* and *yang* organs are paired in an organ system: they perform their functions interdependently and provide each other with energy.

Yin Organs

Heart: The heart, supreme master of the organs, governs the blood and its smooth circulation throughout the body. It houses the Spirit, which is also understood as the capacity to think, remember, comprehend, and respond clearly. The heart holds the capacity for awareness and realization. An individual with an imbalanced heart may experience palpitations, chest pains, poor circulation, poor memory, insomnia, and mental disorders. Bitter herbs help clear cholesterol from the veins and arteries, and affect the heart and meridians. Other herbs, such as zizyphus and biota, calm the Spirit and nurture the heart.

Spleen: This organ assimilates and transports nutrients throughout the body. A weak spleen causes poor digestion, reduced appetite, gas, bloatedness, loose stools, malnutrition, heavy arms and legs, frequent bleeding and bruising, and anemia. Herbs that are tonic, nutritive, sweet, and beneficial to digestion (such as ginseng and wild yam) affect the spleen organ and meridian.

Lungs: Lungs govern respiration and the health of skin and hair. They open to the nose, as well. Lung disorders may manifest themselves in shortness of breath, coughing, difficult breathing, expectoration of mucus, colds, flu, and skin conditions. Pungent herbs (such as cinnamon branches and ephedra) help clear mucus, colds, and the flu, and treat the lung organ and meridians.

Kidneys: The kidneys store Essence, regulate fluid metabolism, dominate the hormonal system of the body, and are connected to the ears. They promote growth, development, reproduction, and a strong immune system. Fertility, sexuality, the urinary system, lowered immunity, lower-back pain, weak knees, edema of the legs, and premature aging are all related to the kidneys. Salty and black-colored herbs, such as rehmannia and *he shou wu*, assist the functions of the kidney organ and meridians.

Liver: This organ stores blood and maintains the smooth flow of *qi*. The liver directly affects the eyes and controls the tendons. It is strongly affected by pressure and emotional stress. Liver imbalances result in spasms, eye ailments, muscle tension, premenstrual syndrome, menstrual irregularities, depression, moodiness, digestive upset, and hypertension. Sour herbs assist the liver, while bitter herbs (such as gentian and gardenia) stimulate the release of bile and calm hypertension.

Yang Organs

Small Intestine: This organ is paired with the heart and assists digestion. The small intestine receives food from the stomach, separates pure fluids from impure ones, transports the pure fluids to various parts of the body, and sends the impure fluids to the large intestine. An imbalance in the small intestine may lead to constipation, diarrhea, and urinary disorders.

Stomach: The stomach is the counterpart of the spleen; it governs digestion. Stomach imbalances result in a lack of appetite, indigestion, vomiting, acid regurgitation, and nausea.

Large Intestine: This organ is paired with the lungs, and is responsible for elimination of waste products. Constipation, dysentery, diarrhea, and hemorrhoids are manifestations of large-intestine disharmony.

Urinary Bladder: The bladder and its partner, the kidneys, store and excrete water. Bladder disharmony results in edema and urinary disorders.

Gallbladder: Partnered with the liver, the gallbladder stores and secretes bile. Traditional Chinese Medicine holds that bile governs a person's decision-making abilities, because it is the only pure substance in the body. Gallbladder imbalances manifest themselves as digestive upset, indecisiveness, timidity, nausea, and belching.

Forms and Uses of Chinese Herbs

*C*hinese herbs come in many forms, including teas, powdered extracts, liquid extracts, pills, tablets, powders, soups, congees, and liniments. Each form has a specific function and purpose, as outlined below.

Forms of Chinese Herbs

Tea is the most assimilable form of Chinese herbs. In this process, herbs (usually dried) are taken and made into tea. Decoction and infusion are two methods of making teas.

Decoctions are made by simmering plant parts in water, until their liquid volume is reduced to three-quarters of the original amount. Two ounces of herbs decocted in four cups of water are cooked when three cups of liquid remain. The decoction process may take 20 to 30 minutes. However, certain herbs (such as gypsum and reishi) must be cooked for up to 60 minutes, so that their properties are properly extracted. Generally, it is appropriate to decoct roots, seeds, barks, twigs, minerals, and leaves in which any of their essential volatile oils are not needed.

Infusions are made by boiling water, pouring it over herbs in a container, and covering the container with a lid. The herbs should stand covered for 10 to 20 minutes. Berries, flowers, and leaves are infused. Herbs with volatile oils, such as mints and cinnamon, should always be infused. Otherwise, their medicinal properties are lost.

Some herbs may be both decocted and infused. Certain leaves and seeds are lightly simmered 10 minutes and then infused for 10 minutes.

It can be difficult to adjust to the taste and smell of Chinese teas. Once an individual becomes accustomed to their smell and taste, however, these teas are quite pleasant to drink.

Standard Dosage: Drink one cup of tea, three times a day.

Powdered extracts are another form of Chinese herbs. In powdered extraction, herbs are cooked in water (at length), and then dried. The drying process occurs either in a dehydrator, or by blowing air over the top of the herb until all liquids have evaporated. The resulting mass is powdered. Volatile oils are caught in a special process and sprayed on the powder. This procedure yields a highly concentrated, medicinal herbal formula, which is well-assimilated by the body. Powdered extracts tend to be more expensive, however, because of the extraction process.

Standard Dosage: Swallow one teaspoonful three times a day, in warm water; or take one standard-size "00" capsule for every 40 pounds of body weight.

Liquid extracts are also highly assimilable by the body. Liquid extraction makes a tincture of the herbs by placing them in alcohol, such as rice wine or red wine, for several minutes. Red wine is preferred in tonics for women, because it replenishes the blood after monthly loss. Some form of sweetener, such as sugar or honey, may be added to form a syrup. Herbs used to promote *qi* and blood circulation are best taken as a wine or tincture, since alcohol effectively carries various substances into the blood. Those who are alcohol-sensitive (such as recovering alcoholics, or individuals with liver congestion or damage), however, should only use alcoholic extracts when added to a cup of boiling water and allowed to cool. This process evaporates most of the alcohol.

Standard Dosage: Swallow one tablespoonful, three times a day.

Pills are a very convenient form of Chinese herbs. Many traditional formulas—called patent medicines—are available in pill-form. They can be found in Chinese pharmacies in major cities, including San Francisco and New York. It takes more metabolic strength to break down pills than it does to assimilate teas. However, pills' lack of taste and their convenience often make them more effective than tea, because individuals are more likely to take them regularly.

Standard Dosage: Take eight pills, three times a day, with warm water. Dosages vary from patent to patent; it is important to follow the specific patent's recommended intake.

Tablets are also available, through Western suppliers of Chinese herbs. Tablets may combine Chinese and Western herbs to create the most effective treatment for certain conditions.

Standard Dosage: Take two tablets three times a day, with warm water.

Powdered herbs are made by grinding dried herbs in a high-speed blender. Powders can be difficult to digest and are, after repeated use, hard on the stomach. Also, powdered herbs quickly lose their potency, because they are exposed to air.

Standard Dosage: One teaspoon three times a day. Alternatively, powdered herbs may be mixed with honey; take one teaspoon three times a day.

Soups are prepared in one of two ways: either by making a tea from the dried herbs for stock, or by cooking herbs in soup water and then adding meat (if desired), grains, beans, and vegetables. Typically, soup herbs are sweet-to-bland in taste and strengthen the body's digestion, energy, and blood. Many of these herbs are left in the soup and consumed with it. Astragalus, codonopsis, dioscorea (or Chinese wild yam), jujube dates, lycii berries, and reishi mushrooms are often added to soup. For a list of soup recipes, refer to the chapter entitled "Chinese Herbal Diet."

Standard Dosage: Eat a normal, meal-size quantity of soup, one to three times a day.

Congees, which consist of herbs cooked with food, are similar to soups. To make a congee, however, herbs are cooked at length with sweet rice until the herbs and grain take on a porridge consistency. Congees are highly assimilable and nutritious. They are particularly appropriate for individuals convalescing from a long-term illness, operation, or childbirth; or for people with severely debilitating diseases, lowered immunity or energy, or extremely poor digestion.

Herbs used in soups are also used in congees; these herbs strengthen certain organs or bodily systems, as well as the body's overall *qi*, blood, and immunity. For a list of congee recipes, refer to the chapter entitled "Chinese Herbal Diet."

Standard Dosage: Eat a normal, meal-size quantity of congee, one to three times a day.

Liniments are made through the same process as tinctures are created. Since liniments are for external use only, however, cheaper rubbing alcohol is used. Liniments are used to treat sprains, bruises, muscle and joint pain, and injuries. They generally contain warm, circulating herbs such as angelica, cayenne, cloves, ginger, myrrh, and wild ginger. Rub or massage this form of herbal treatment on the affected area.

Herbal Dosages

Proper herbal dosage is crucial. A sufficient quantity of herbs must be taken in order for the treatment to be effective. Quite often, people ingest the proper herbs or formulas, but don't experience desired results, simply because they are not taking a sufficient herbal dosage. On the other hand, it is possible to take too many herbs. Ingesting an excessive amount of herbs over a long period of time can injure the digestive tract and impair the body's ability to break down and absorb food.

Chinese herbs generally yield a slow, progressive improvement, as opposed to the quick cure most Westerners expect. However, Chinese herbal treatments effect lasting changes, and don't create further imbalances or produce side effects if properly used.

Most herbs should be taken warm, either by drinking warm teas, or by swallowing pills, powders, capsules, tablets, or extracts with warm water. Warm water facilitates the assimilation of herbs and protects the digestive system.

The standard dosage for Chinese herbs is an average of 3 to 9 grams, or 1/9 to 1/3 ounce. A formula may consist of up to 200 grams (or 8 ounces) of herbs, and may include as many as 20 herbs. Generally, formulas are taken three times a day. Dosages vary according to body weight, age, and the severity of a particular condition. Heavier bodies need a higher dosage, and lighter bodies need a smaller dosage.

Following is a Chinese-formula dosage chart, according to age. These guide-lines apply to individuals of average weight, height, and sensitivity. Dosage adjustments should be made according to individual weight, height, and sensitivity.

DOSAGE GUIDELINES	
Age	Fractional Adult Dosage
0 to 1 year	1/10 to 1/75 of adult dosage
2 to 6 years	1/8 to 1/10 of adult dosage
6 to 12 years	1/3 to 1/2 of adult dosage
12 to 15 years	1/2 to 2/3 of adult dosage
15 to 70 years	full, adult dosage
over 70 years	1/2 of adult dosage

When to Take Herbs

Empty Stomach: Individuals with a watery condition accompanied by mucus, or who wish to detoxify, should take herbs on an empty stomach. Herbs taken on an empty stomach have a more potent effect.

Before Meals: Treatment of nervous diseases, intestinal issues, and fat reduction are best accomplished by taking herbs before meals. Tonics are most effective when taken before meals.

After Meals: Treatment of gas, indigestion, lung conditions, sinus ailments, and mucus prevention are best accomplished by taking herbs after meals.

Mixed with Food: Herbs mixed with food act as a tonic; they are also effective in the treatment of weak individuals or digestive disturbances.

Between Meals: Urinary and nervous disorders are most effectively treated by taking herbs between meals.

Processing Herbs

The processing methods developed by Traditional Chinese Medicine reduce herbal toxicity, increase herbs' therapeutic effectiveness, alter their properties, and remove offending odors. Some formulas call for processed herbs, such as dried, fried ginger, or honey-fried licorice. Herbs can be purchased in various forms from Chinese pharmacies and herb suppliers.

Steamed and Dried: Some herbs, such as *Rehmannia glutinosa*, are steamed and dried; this process changes the herb's energy from cool to warm.

Dry-Roasted or Stir-Fried: These processes increase herbs' heating energies. Ginger is frequently dry-roasted by toasting it in a dry pan. Licorice and astragalus are often stir-fried with honey, which boosts their ability to effectively treat the digestive system.

Spirits or Wine: Herbs may also be soaked in grain spirits or wine; the resulting compounds are called liquid extracts. Liquid extracts quickly enter the blood and have an ascending energy. Deer antlers and *dong quai* are frequently prepared as liquid extracts.

Salt Processing: Herbs processed with salt become tonics for the urinary tract. This process also enhances a formula's descending action.

Vinegar Processing: Since the sour taste goes to the liver, the effectiveness of herbs processed with sour substances (such as vinegar) is carried to that organ. The sour taste also has a descending and contracting energy.

Baking: Herbs baked with honey become tonic and moistening; herbs baked with ginger become warming and dispersing, and promote circulation.

Considerations in Herbal Administration

• Use high-quality, fresh herbs whenever possible.

• Herbs with strong therapeutic actions (such as diaphoretics and purgatives) should be used with great care when administered to severely weakened individuals.

• Strong, blood-moving herbs (such as emmenagogues and purgatives with a strong downward action) should not be administered to pregnant women, since they cause miscarriages and abortions.

• If an acute disease and a chronic disease occur simultaneously, the acute disease should be treated first, with fewer herbs used in the formula. Small doses should be taken every one or two hours; frequency of dosage should taper off as symptoms subside. Acute diseases should improve within one to three days, at most. If they do not, the herbal treatment should be reevaluated.

• Chronic diseases should be treated slowly and gently, with a formula balanced in energies and properties, and the formulation administered over a prolonged period of time. Herbal formulas should be taken three times daily. Calculate the number of years since the inception of the condition, and continue the treatment for an equal number of months. Chronic diseases should improve within two weeks. If they do not, the herbal treatment should be reevaluated.

• Excessively cooling and bitter herbs should not be taken frequently, or over a prolonged period of time. These herbs can damage the digestive system.

• Excessively heating herbs should rarely be used in summer, while cold-natured herbs with strong eliminative properties should rarely be used in winter. Fasting and detoxification are best practiced during the spring and fall.

• Rapid recovery from skin diseases and disorders of the throat, vagina, rectum, eyes, ears, and nose may be facilitated by fomentations, gargles, douches, boluses, herbal enemas, suppositories, and eye- and eardrops. Respiratory conditions benefit from the application of syrups and herbal vapor inhalations.

• Infants and small children may be treated with herbal baths and fomentations. Young children can be given powdered herbs mixed with honey to form a paste.

Common Chinese Herbs

The following herbs are a select representation of the hundreds of herbs used in Chinese medicine. They are listed by their common, Latin, and Mandarin Chinese names; parts used; energy; taste; affinity (organs/meridians affected and therapeutic action); most common uses; and dosages. Contraindications are included where appropriate. For clarification of any of the following terms, refer to the Glossary, on page 182.

Acanthopanax

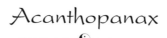

Acanthopanax gracilistylus
Wu Jia Pi

Part used: root bark
Energy and taste: warm; pungent and bitter
Affinity: kidneys, liver; antirheumatic
Uses: This herb (a close relative of Siberian ginseng) treats conditions associated with aging, such as rheumatism, arthritis, soft sinews and bones, urinary difficulty, edema, swollen legs. It is also effective in dealing with developmental delays in children's motor functions.

Precautions: Do not use this herb in the presence of deficient heat.

Dosage: Use 4.5 to 15 grams of the herb in a decoction. Generally, *wu jia pi* is soaked in rice wine and taken in daily teaspoon doses.

Achyranthes

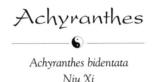

Achyranthes bidentata
Niu Xi

Part used: root

Energy and taste: neutral; bitter, sour

Affinity: liver, kidneys; moves blood

Uses: Achyranthes treats menstrual pain, amenorrhea, pain in the lower back and knees, painful urination accompanied by kidney stones, bloody urine, vaginal discharge, sore throats, nosebleeds, bloody vomit, toothaches, bleeding gums, dizziness, headaches, and blurred vision.

Precautions: Do not use this herb during pregnancy, since it could cause miscarriage. Also, achyranthes may aggravate diarrhea, excessive menstruation, and spermatorrhea.

Dosage: decoction, 9 to 15 grams

Aconite

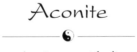

Aconitum carmichaeli
Fu Zi

Part used: prepared root of Szechwan aconite

Energy and taste: hot; pungent, toxic

Affinity: heart, kidney, spleen; warms the interior

Uses: Aconite alleviates coldness, pain, and diarrhea; and helps to break down undigested food in the stools. It is a potent metabolic stimulant, widely used to counteract all cold conditions.

Precautions: Do not use aconite in the presence of pregnancy and deficient heat; or with fritillary, trichosanthes, or pinellia. This herb is generally prepared with salt and vinegar, which reduce its toxicity.

Dosage: Decoct 1.5 to 9 grams. This herb is toxic: use prepared aconite only. It must be boiled for 30 to 60 minutes before other herbs are added.

Note: Aconite tea's toxicity has not been adequately neutralized if it causes a numbing sensation in the mouth; if such a sensation occurs, the tea should not be used. Consumption of mung beans is the antidote for aconite poisoning.

Agastache

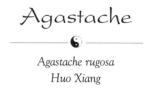

Agastache rugosa
Huo Xiang

Part used: leaf
Energy and taste: slightly warm; pungent
Affinity: lungs, spleen, and stomach; aromatic stomachic
Uses: Agastache treats indigestion, abdominal distension, nausea, vomiting, reduced appetite, morning sickness, summer colds and flu, and diarrhea.
Precautions: Do not use this herb if heat in the stomach or deficient heat are present.
Dosage: Decoct 4.5 to 9 grams for no more than 15 minutes.

Alismatis

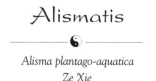

Alisma plantago-aquatica
Ze Xie

Part used: water plantain rhizome
Energy and taste: cold; sweet, bland
Affinity: kidneys, bladder; diuretic
Uses: Alismatis is effective in the treatment of urinary difficulty, edema, diarrhea, abdominal bloating, diabetes, nephritis, cystitis, and kidney stones. It is a useful diuretic for the weak and elderly.

Precautions: Do not use in the presence of spermatorrhea, vaginal discharge, or coldness.

Dosage: decoction, 6 to 15 grams

Alpinia

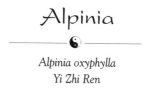

Alpinia oxyphylla
Yi Zhi Ren

Part used: fruit of black cardamom
Energy and taste: warm; pungent
Affinity: kidney, spleen; tonifies *yang*
Uses: Alpinia is used to treat urinary incontinence, frequent and copious urination, dribbling of urine, diarrhea, abdominal pain, excessive salivation, and vomiting.
Precautions: Spermatorrhea; frequent or scant dark-yellow urination; and yellow vaginal discharge with odor can be aggravated by use of this herb.
Dosage: Decoct 3 to 9 grams of crushed alpinia.

Alum

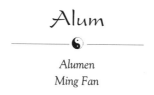

Alumen
Ming Fan

Part used: mineral
Energy and taste: cold; sour, astringent
Affinity: large intestine, liver, lungs, spleen, stomach; topical application
Uses: Alum may alleviate a swollen, painful throat; swollen, painful eyes; jaundice; chronic diarrhea; bloody stools; bleeding gums; bleeding hemorrhoids; uterine bleeding; and vaginal discharge. Used as an external wash, alum kills parasites such as ringworm and scabies.
Precautions: Internal use of *ming fan* should be administered cautiously. Do not use this herb in the presence of weak digestion.
Dosage: Crush 3 to 5 grams of alum; make the herb into a paste for topical use.

American Ginseng

Panax quinquefolium
Xi Yang Shen

Part used: root
Energy and taste: cold; sweet, slightly bitter
Affinity: heart, kidneys, lungs; tonifies *yin*
Uses: American ginseng successfully counteracts chronic, low-grade fevers, weakness, post-fever irritability and thirst, wheezing, expectoration of blood, and loss of voice. It also moistens the *yin*.
Precautions: Since American ginseng is a cooling herb, it may aggravate diarrhea and poor digestion.
Dosage: decoction, 2.4 to 9 grams

Anemarrhena

Anemarrhena asphodeloides
Zhi Mu

Part used: rhizomes and stems
Energy and taste: cold; bitter
Affinity: lungs, stomach, kidneys; clears heat
Uses: Anemarrhena treats high fever; irritability; thirst; coughing accompanied by the expectoration of thick, yellow phlegm; night sweats; bleeding gums; spermatorrhea; nocturnal emissions; and oral ulcers.
Precautions: Do not use this herb in the presence of loose stools or diarrhea.
Dosage: decoction, 6 to 12 grams

Angelica

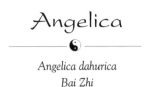

Angelica dahurica
Bai Zhi

Part used: Chinese angelica root
Energy and taste: warm; pungent
Affinity: lungs, stomach; treats the exterior
Uses: *Angelica dahurica* counteracts migraine and lesser headaches, nasal congestion, pain above the eyes, sores and carbuncles in the early stages of development, and vaginal discharge.
Precautions: Do not use this herb to treat individuals with anemia or deficient heat.
Dosage: decoction, 3 to 9 grams

Apricot Seed

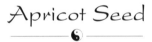

Prunus armeniaca
Xing Ren

Part used: seed
Energy and taste: slightly warm, slightly toxic; bitter
Affinity: large intestine, lungs; stops coughing and wheezing
Uses: Apricot seed treats various coughs, whether caused by heat or cold; it is particularly effective in counteracting dry coughs. It is also used in the treatment of wheezing, bronchitis, and asthma, and as a mild laxative.
Precautions: Do not use this herb with astragalus, pueraria, or scute; to treat infants; or if diarrhea is present.
Dosage: Chop the seeds before the decocting process. Use 3 to 9 grams and decoct for 10 minutes only.

Areca

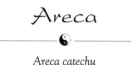

Areca catechu
Bing Lang

Part used: betel nut (seed)
Energy and taste: warm; pungent, bitter
Affinity: large intestine, stomach; parasiticide
Uses: Areca eliminates intestinal parasites (particularly tapeworms), food congestion, abdominal bloating, and constipation.
Precautions: Do not use areca in the presence of poor digestion or organ prolapse.
Dosage: Use 6 to 12 grams of decoction; 60 to 120 grams are appropriate when areca is used alone to treat tapeworms. The decoction should be consumed when cool, to reduce side effects. For best results, soak the seeds a few hours before decocting.

Asparagus

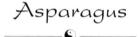

Asparagus cochinchinensis
Tian Men Dong

Part used: tuber of Chinese asparagus
Energy and taste: very cold; sweet, bitter
Affinity: kidneys, lungs; tonifies *yin*
Uses: Chinese asparagus tuber treats dry mouth; thick, blood-streaked mucus; dry coughing; tuberculosis; mouth sores; low-grade, afternoon fevers; constipation due to dryness; and thirst.
Precautions: Avoid use of this herb in the presence of loss of appetite, diarrhea, and coughing accompanied by clear-to-white phlegm.
Dosage: decoction, 6 to 15 grams

Astragalus

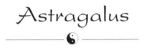

Astragalus membranaceus
Huang Qi

Part used: root
Energy and taste: slightly warm; sweet
Affinity: lungs, spleen; tonifies energy
Uses: Astragalus relieves lack of appetite; fatigue; diarrhea; prolapse of the uterus, stomach, or rectum; uterine bleeding caused by weakness; spontaneous or excessive sweating; shortness of breath; frequent colds or flu; postpartum fever, caused by loss of blood and energy; symptoms associated with a severe loss of blood; and edema. It also helps heal undrained sores and wounds that are slow to heal, numbness of limbs, and paralysis.
Precautions: congestion of any sort, deficient heat, excess heat, skin lesions
Dosage: decoction, 9 to 30 grams

Atractylodis

Atractylodes macrocephala
Bai Zhu

Part used: rhizome
Energy and taste: warm; bitter, sweet
Affinity: spleen, stomach; tonifies energy
Uses: Atractylodis is used to stop diarrhea, fatigue, lack of appetite, vomiting, edema, involuntary sweating caused by low energy, and restless fetal movment.
Precautions: Do not use this herb in the presence of deficient heat.
Dosage: decoction, 4.5 to 9 grams

Biota

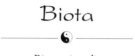

Biota orientalis
Bai Zi Ren

Part used: seeds
Energy and taste: neutral; sweet
Affinity: heart, kidneys, large intestine; calmative
Uses: Biota treats insomnia; irritability; forgetfulness; palpitations accompanied by anxiety; constipation in the elderly, debilitated, and postpartum women; and night sweats.
Precautions: Do not used biota if loose stools or phlegm are present, or with chrysanthemum.
Dosage: decoction, 6 to 18 grams

Black Pepper

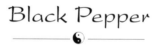

Piper nigrum
Hu Jiao

Part used: the fruits
Energy and taste: hot; pungent
Affinity: large intestine, stomach; warms interior
Uses: Black pepper can be used to counteract vomiting, diarrhea, abdominal pain, clear-to-white lung mucus, coldness, indigestion, food congestion, and poor circulation.
Precautions: Avoid use of black pepper in the presence of deficient heat.
Dosage: decoction or powdered, 1.5 to 4.5 grams

Bupleurum

———— ☯ ————

Bupleurum chinesis, B. scorponeraefolium
Chai Hu

Part used: root of hare's ear
Energy and taste: cool; pungent, bitter
Affinity: liver, gallbladder; treats the exterior
Uses: Bupleurum treats colds, alternating chills and fever, malarial fever, irritability, vomiting, hepatitis, cirrhosis and other liver disorders, dizziness, irregular menstruation, premenstrual syndrome, depression, and organ prolapse.
Precautions: This herb is very drying—it should not be used in long-term treatment or if there is weakness, anemia, or deficient heat present. Bupleurum should always be combined with *dang gui* or lycii berries, since these herbs moisten and strengthen the blood, and counteract bupleurum's drying action.
Dosage: decoction, 3 to 12 grams

Burdock

———— ☯ ————

Arctium lappa
Niu Bang Zi

Part used: seeds
Energy and taste: cold; pungent, bitter
Affinity: lungs, stomach; treats the exterior
Uses: Burdock seeds treat swollen, red, sore throats; fever; coughing; pneumonia; bronchitis; lung congestion; measles (in its early stages); skin lesions; boils; juvenile chicken pox; and smallpox.
Precautions: Avoid using this herb in the presence of open sores, or during the later stages of measles.
Dosage: decoction, 3 to 9 grams

Cardamom

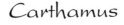

Amomum villosum
Sha Ren

Part used: seeds
Energy and taste: warm; pungent
Affinity: spleen, stomach; aromatic stomachic
Uses: Cardamom can be used to treat vomiting, nausea, abdominal pain, loss of appetite, indigestion, chronic diarrhea, morning sickness, and restless fetal movement.
Precautions: Do not use cardamom in the presence of deficient heat.
Dosage: Decoct 1.5 to 6 grams of cardamom for 10 minutes (maximum); add it near the end of the decoction process, while cooking other herbs.

Carthamus

Carthamus tinctorius
Hong Hua

Part used: safflower flower
Energy and taste: warm; pungent
Affinity: heart, liver; moves blood
Uses: Safflower is used to treat delayed menses, poor blood circulation, blood clots, lower abdominal pains, amenorrhea, postpartum dizziness, and abdominal masses. It also stops bleeding and pain from wounds, and the incomplete expression of rashes and measles.
Precautions: Do not use safflower during pregnancy.
Dosage: Decoct safflower for five minutes. Dosages should include 3 to 9 grams of the herb.

Chaenomeles

Chaenomeles lagenaria
Mu Gua

Part used: Chinese quince fruit
Energy and taste: slightly warm; sour
Affinity: liver, spleen; antirheumatic
Uses: Chaenomeles can be used to counteract leg cramps, edema, tendon and muscle spasms, indigestion, diarrhea, vomiting, and weakness of the lower back and legs.
Precautions: Excessive use of this herb can harm teeth and bones. Do not use chaenomeles while colds or fever are present.
Dosage: decoction, 4.5 to 12 grams

Chrysanthemum

Chrysanthemum morifolium
Ju Hua

Part used: flowers
Energy and taste: slightly cold; pungent, sweet, bitter
Affinity: lungs, liver; treats the exterior
Uses: Chrysanthemum relieves fever; headaches; dizziness; skin eruptions; red, painful, dry, and swollen eyes; excessive eye tearing; spots in the field of vision; and blurry vision, due to kidney and liver dysfunctions. This herb can be used with honeysuckle to alleviate high blood pressure.
Dosage: infusion, 5 to 15 grams

Cimicifuga

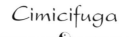

Cimicifuga foetida
Sheng Ma

Part used: rhizome of Chinese black cohosh
Energy and taste: cool; sweet, pungent
Affinity: large intestine, lungs, spleen, stomach; treats the exterior
Uses: Chinese black cohosh may alleviate colds, flu, early stages of measles, sore teeth, painful gums, ulcerated lips, canker sores, swollen and painful throat, shortness of breath, fatigue, and prolapse caused by lack of energy.
Precautions: Avoid use of Chinese black cohosh in the presence of deficient heat.
Dosage: decoction, 1.5 to 9 gm

Cinnamon Bark

Cinnamomum cassiae
Rou Gui

Part used: inner bark of the tree
Energy and taste: hot; pungent, sweet
Affinity: heart, kidneys, liver, spleen; warms interior
Uses: Cinnamon bark alleviates an aversion to cold, cold limbs, weak back, impotence, frequent urination, abdominal pain and spasms caused by coldness, reduced appetite, diarrhea, wheezing, and rheumatism caused by coldness. This herb also improves digestion.
Precautions: Do not use this herb in the presence of deficient heat, excessive heat, bleeding caused by heat, or pregnancy.
Dosage: Cinnamon bark is usually taken as powder or pill, since decoction causes a loss of volatile oils. If this herb is decocted, prepare it for five minutes (maximum); crush it into small pieces. Use 1.5 to 4.5 grams of cinnamon bark.

Cinnamon Twig

Cinnamomum cassiae

Gui Zhi

Part used: twig

Energy and taste: warm; pungent, sweet

Affinity: heart, lungs, bladder; treats the exterior

Uses: Cinnamon twigs alleviate colds; flu; fever; shoulder, joint, limb, and abdominal pain; edema; weakness of the heart; and muscular contractions. It also warms the hands.

Dosage: Cinnamon twigs should be prepared as an infusion: Use 3 to 9 grams for exterior conditions, or 9 to 15 grams for pain.

Cistanches

Cistanche deserticola

Rou Cong Rong

Part used: fleshy stem of the broomrape

Energy and taste: warm; sweet, salty

Affinity: large intestine, kidneys; tonifies *yang*

Uses: Cistanches can be used to treat impotence; spermatorrhea; urinary incontinence; posturinary dripping; cold-induced pains in the lower back and knees; excessive uterine bleeding; infertility; white vaginal discharge; and constipation from dryness, especially in the elderly and those with weakness or anemia.

Precautions: Do not use this herb in the presence of deficient heat or diarrhea characterized by weak digestion.

Dosage: decoction, 9 to 21 grams

Clematis

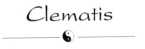

Clematis chinensis
Wei Ling Xian

Part used: root and stem of Chinese clematis
Energy and taste: warm; pungent, salty
Affinity: bladder; antirheumatic
Uses: Clematis can alleviate arthritis, rheumatism, and stiffness.
Precautions: Avoid use of this herb in the presence of *qi* or blood deficiencies.
Dosage: decoction, 6 to 12 grams

Codonopsis

Codonopsis pilosula
Dang Shen

Part used: root
Energy and taste: neutral; sweet
Affinity: lungs, spleen; tonifies energy
Uses: This herb can treat lack of appetite; indigestion; fatigue; weak or tired limbs; diarrhea; vomiting; prolapse of the uterus, stomach, or rectum; chronic coughing; shortness of breath; and expectoration of copious, white-to-clear mucus.
Dosage: decoction, 9 to 30 grams

Coix

Coix lachryma jobi
Yi Yi Ren

Part used: Chinese barley seeds (Job's tears)
Energy and taste: slightly cold; bland, sweet

Affinity: spleen, lungs, kidneys; diuretic

Uses: Coix is effective in the treatment of edema, urinary difficulty, swelling of the legs, diarrhea, skin eruptions accompanied by pus, and chronic spasms. It also increases joint mobility.

Precautions: Because of its diuretic nature, exercise caution when using this herb during pregnancy.

Dosage: Cook coix and consume it as food, or use 9 to 30 grams of it in a decoction.

Coltsfoot

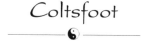

Tussilago farfara
Kuan Dong Hua

Part used: flower

Energy and taste: warm; pungent

Affinity: lungs; expectorant

Uses: Coltsfoot is a specific for coughing and wheezing, bronchitis, shortness of breath, and hoarseness.

Precautions: This herb should not be used in the presence of heat conditions, or with fritillaria, magnolia flowers, ephedra, scute, coptis, or astragalus.

Dosage: infusion, 1.5 to 9 grams

Coptis

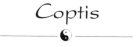

Coptis chinensis
Huang Lian

Part used: rhizome

Energy and taste: cold; bitter

Affinity: heart, large intestine, liver, stomach; clears heat and dampness

Uses: Coptis can alleviate high fever; irritability; disorientation; delirium; painful, red eyes; a sore throat; boils; carbuncles; abscesses; vomiting; acid regurgitation; insomnia; nosebleeds; bloody urine, stools, or vomit; and bad breath. It also clears damp heat.

Precautions: Do not use coptis in the presence of deficient heat, coldness, loose stools, or diarrhea. Long-term use of this herb can injure the digestion.

Dosage: decoction, 1.5 to 9 grams

Cornus

Cornus officinalis
Shan Zhu Yu

Part used: Asiatic Cornelian cherry fruit
Energy and taste: slightly warm; sour
Affinity: kidneys, liver; astringent
Uses: Cornus can relieve excessive urination; incontinence; spermatorrhea; excessive sweating, particularly from shock; light-headedness; dizziness; soreness and weakness of the lower back and knees; impotence; excessive uterine bleeding; prolonged menstruation; night sweats; hearing loss; and tinnitus.

Precautions: Do not use cornus when painful and difficult urination are present, or with platycodon or siler.

Dosage: Prepare 3 to 12 grams of cornus as a decoction; to treat shock, use 30 to 60 grams of the herb.

Corydalis

Corydalis yanhusuo
Yan Hu Suo

Part used: rhizome
Energy and taste: warm; pungent, bitter
Affinity: heart, liver, lungs, stomach; moves blood
Uses: This herb can be used to treat menstrual, chest, and abdominal pain; pain caused by traumatic injury; hernia pain; and migraines. Corydalis is one

of the most effective herbs for the treatment of pain.

Precautions: Do not use this herb during pregnancy; its strong blood-moving action could cause miscarriage.

Dosage: decoction, 4.5 to 12 grams

Curcuma

———— ☯ ————

Curcuma longa
Yu Jin

Part used: turmeric tuber
Energy and taste: cool; pungent, bitter
Affinity: heart, lungs, liver; moves blood
Uses: Turmeric tuber is used to treat pain resulting from traumatic injury; chest, abdominal, side, or menstrual pain; liver congestion; anxiety; agitation; seizures; mental disturbance and confusion; jaundice; and hepatitis.
Precautions: Do not use curcuma tuber in the presence of deficient heat, or during pregnancy.
Dosage: decoction, 4.5 to 9 grams

Cuscuta

———— ☯ ————

Cuscuta chinensis
Tu Si Zi

Part used: Chinese dodder seeds
Energy and taste: neutral; pungent, sweet
Affinity: kidneys, liver; tonifies *yang*
Uses: Cuscuta may alleviate impotence; nocturnal emissions; premature ejaculation; tinnitus; frequent urination; sore back muscles; vaginal discharge; dizziness; blurred vision; the appearance of spots in the field of vision; diarrhea, or loose stools; lack of appetite; the movement of a restless fetus; and impending miscarriage. It also strengthens tendons and bones.

Precautions: Do not use this herb in the presence of deficient heat, constipation, or scant and dark urine.
Dosage: decoction, 9 to 15 grams

Cyperus

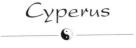

Cyperus rotundus
Xiang Fu

Part used: rhizome of sedge plant
Energy and taste: neutral; pungent, slightly bitter, slightly sweet
Affinity: liver; regulates energy
Uses: Cyperus can be used to relieve pain in the ribs and chest, upper abdominal distension, menstrual disorders, painful or irregular menstruation, depression, moodiness, menstrual cramps, indigestion, gas, and nausea.
Precautions: Avoid use of this herb in the presence of weakness, fatigue, or deficient heat. It is a very drying herb.
Dosage: decoction, 4.5 to 12 grams

Dandelion

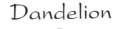

Taraxacum mongolicum
Pu Gong Ying

Part used: root
Energy and taste: cold; bitter, sweet
Affinity: liver, stomach; clears heat and toxins
Uses: Dandelion is used in the treatment of red, swollen, and painful eyes; hard abscesses and sores; breast abscesses; jaundice; and painful urination. This herb also promotes lactation.
Precautions: An overdose of dandelion can cause mild diarrhea.
Dosage: decoction, 9 to 30 grams

Dang Gui

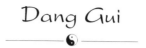

Angelica sinensis
Dang Gui

Part used: Chinese angelica root, also known as *tang kuei*
Energy and taste: warm; sweet, pungent, bitter
Affinity: heart, liver, spleen; tonifies blood
Uses: *Dang gui* strengthens the blood and regulates menses. It is useful in the treatment of anemia; constipation due to anemia; all gynecological problems, including irregular menstruation, amenorrhea, and dysmenorrhea; tinnitus; blurred vision; palpitations; abdominal pain; pain resulting from traumatic injury; dry skin; and skin eruptions.
Precautions: Avoid use of this herb in the presence of diarrhea or deficient heat.
Dosage: decoction, 3 to 15 grams

Dendrobium

Dendrobium nobile
Shi Hu

Part used: above ground portion
Energy and taste: cold; sweet, slightly salty, bland
Affinity: kidneys, stomach; tonifies *yin*
Uses: Dendrobium alleviates a parched mouth, severe thirst, dry heaves, mouth sores, weakness resulting from prolonged fever, and poor eyesight. It also strengthens the lower back.
Precautions: Do not use this herb during the early stages of colds or flu, or in the presence of abdominal distension.
Dosage: decoction, 6 to 15 grams

Dianthus

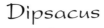

Dianthus superbus, D. chinensis
Qu Mai

Part used: parts of "pinks" carnations that grow above ground
Energy and taste: cold; bitter
Affinity: bladder, heart, small intestine
Uses: Dianthus treats painful urination, urinary-tract infections, bloody urination, constipation, and amenorrhea caused by stagnant blood.
Precautions: Use of dianthus during pregnancy, or in the presence of spleen or kidney deficiency, is prohibited.
Dosage: decoction, 6 to 12 grams and up to 24 grams

Dipsacus

Dipsacus asper
Xu Duan

Part used: Japanese teasel root
Energy and taste: slightly warm; bitter, pungent
Affinity: kidneys, liver; tonifies *yang*
Uses: Dipsacus is used in the treatment of lower-back and knee pain, stiff joints, uterine bleeding, vaginal discharge, bleeding during pregnancy, impending miscarriage, and pain caused by traumatic injuries. This herb will also calm a fetus.
Dosage: decoction, 6 to 21 grams

Eclipta

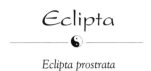

Eclipta prostrata
Han Lian Cao

Part used: entirety of the plant
Energy and taste: cool; sweet, sour
Affinity: kidneys, liver; tonifies *yin*
Uses: Eclipta can relieve dizziness; blurred vision; vertigo; premature graying of the hair; bloody vomit, expectoration, stools, or urine; uterine bleeding; nosebleeds; and tinnitus.
Precautions: Do not use this herb in the presence of poor digestion or diarrhea.
Dosage: decoction, 9 to 15 grams of dry herb or 30 grams of fresh herb

Ephedra

Ephedra spp.
Ma Huang

Part used: parts that grow above ground
Energy and taste: warm; pungent, slightly bitter
Affinity: lungs, bladder; treats the exterior
Uses: Ephedra is used to treat colds accompanied by chills, slight fevers, headaches, absence of sweating, asthmatic wheezing, and rheumatic complaints accompanied by water retention.
Precautions: This herb can raise blood pressure. Do not use ephedra in the presence of hypertension; *yin* deficiencies, including weakness and deficient heat; or insomnia. Extensive use of this herb can cause heavy sweating and weaken the body. Please note that certain products use this herb to stimulate energy; this use of ephedra is dangerous, and should be avoided.
Dosage: decoction, 3 to 9 grams

Epimedium

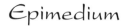

Epimedium grandiflorum
Yin Yang Huo

Part used: parts that grow above ground
Energy and taste: warm; pungent, sweet
Affinity: kidneys, liver; tonifies *yang*
Uses: Epimedium is useful in the treatment of impotence; frigidity; spermatorrhea; frequent urination; forgetfulness; withdrawal from chemical addiction; painful, cold lower backs and knees; spasms or cramps in the hands and feet; joint pain; numbness of limbs; dizziness; and menstrual irregularity. It also helps to repair bone fractures.
Precautions: Do not use epimedium in the presence of deficient heat, or for prolonged periods of time: it can cause dizziness, vomiting, dry mouth, thirst, and nosebleeds.
Dosage: infusion, 6 to 15 grams

Eucommia

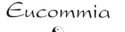

Eucommia ulmoides
Du Zhong

Part used: bark
Energy and taste: warm; sweet, slightly pungent
Affinity: kidneys, liver; tonifies *yang*
Uses: Eucommia may alleviate weakness and pain in the lower back and knees, fatigue, frequent urination, bleeding during pregnancy, impending miscarriage, hypertension, premature aging, and impotence. It also strengthens tendons and bones, and can calm a restless fetus.
Precautions: This herb's heating nature can aggravate deficient heat.
Dosage: decoction, 6 to 15 grams

Fennel

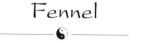

Foeniculum vulgare
Xiao Hui Xiang

Part used: seeds
Energy and taste: warm; pungent
Affinity: liver, kidneys, spleen, stomach; warms interior
Uses: Fennel may prevent indigestion, gas, bloatedness, spasms of gastrointestinal tract, cold-induced abdominal pain, reduced appetite, and vomiting.
Precautions: deficient heat
Dosage: Eat fennel directly, or decoct 3 to 9 grams of this herb for 5 minutes.

Forsythia

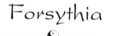

Forsythia suspensa
Lian Qiao

Part used: fruit
Energy and taste: cool; bitter, slightly pungent
Affinity: heart, liver, gallbladder; clears heat and toxins
Uses: Forsythia is used to treat skin, throat, mouth, gum, and skin inflammations; high fever accompanied by thirst; lymphatic swelling; and neck lumps.
Precautions: Avoid using this herb in the presence of poor digestion accompanied by diarrhea.
Dosage: decoction, 6 to 15 grams

Fritillary

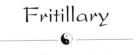

Fritillaria thunbergii
Zhe Bei Mu

Part used: bulb
Energy and taste: cold; bitter
Affinity: heart, lungs; clears phlegm and stops coughing
Uses: Fritillary can be effective in the treatment of bronchitis; bronchial asthma; coughs accompanied by thick, yellow phlegm; hard lymphatic lumps; breast lumps and swellings; and thyroid tumors.
Precautions: Do not use this herb if low energy, poor digestion, or coldness are present.
Dosage: decoction, 3 to 9 grams

Gambir

Uncaria rhynchophylla
Gou Teng

Part used: stems and thorns of hook vine
Energy and taste: cool; sweet
Affinity: heart, liver; extinguishes wind, relieves spasms
Uses: Gambir can alleviate tremors, spasms, seizures, headaches, irritability, redness of eyes, dizziness, hypertension, fever, and convulsions.
Dosage: Decoct 6 to 15 grams of gambir for no more than 10 minutes.

Gardenia

Gardenia jasminoides
Zhi Zi

Part used: fruit
Energy and taste: cold; bitter

Affinity: heart, liver, lungs, stomach; clears heat
Uses: Gardenia treats irritability, fever, restlessness, insomnia, painful urination, jaundice, hepatitis, hypertension, depression, ulcers, and redness of eyes.
Precautions: Avoid use of this herb in the presence of loose stools or loss of appetite.
Dosage: Crush 3 to 12 grams of gardenia, then decoct the herb.

Garlic

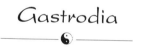

Allium sativum
Da Suan

Part used: bulb
Energy and taste: warm; pungent
Affinity: large intestine, lungs, spleen, stomach; parasiticide
Uses: Garlic eliminates intestinal parasites, such as hookworms and pinworms; yeast and fungus; diarrhea; dysentery; flu; and lung complaints, including bronchitis, pneumonia, and coughing accompanied by copious white phlegm.
Precautions: Do not use this herb in the presence of deficient heat.
Dosage: decoction, 6 to 15 grams or 3 to 5 cloves

Gastrodia

Gastrodia elata
Tian Ma

Part used: rhizome
Energy and taste: neutral; sweet
Affinity: liver; extinguishes wind, relieves spasms
Uses: Gastrodia can alleviate spasms; tremors; headaches, including migraines; dizziness; pediatric convulsions; epilepsy; tetany; hemiplegia; and numbness of the lower back and extremities.
Dosage: decoction, 3 to 9 grams

Gentian

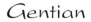

Gentiana spp.
Long Dan Cao

Part used: Chinese gentian root
Energy and taste: cold; bitter
Affinity: gallbladder, liver, stomach; clears damp heat
Uses: Gentian is used to treat red, swollen, and sore throats; red, swollen, and sore eyes; swollen and painful ears; sudden deafness; jaundice; genital pain or swelling; foul-smelling vaginal discharge; vaginal itching; and infantile convulsions.
Precautions: poor digestion with diarrhea
Dosage: decoction, 3 to 9 grams

Ginger, Dried

Zingiber officinale
Gan Jiang

Part used: dried root
Energy and taste: hot; pungent
Affinity: heart, lungs, spleen, stomach; warms interior
Uses: Dried ginger is effective in the treatment of coldness, an aversion to cold, diarrhea, nausea, vomiting, coughing accompanied by white phlegm, gas, bloating, and spasms and cramps caused by coldness. This herb also promotes healthy menses and improves digestion.
Precautions: deficient heat, bleeding from heat, pregnancy
Dosage: *Gan jiang* is usually taken in powder or pill form; decoction causes a loss of volatile oils. Use 3 to 12 grams of this herb.
Note: Fresh ginger, or *sheng jiang*, is also used. It is a specific for colds, flu, coughing accompanied by white phlegm, and vomiting. Infuse 3 to 9 grams of *sheng jiang*. Avoid use of this herb in the presence of yellow phlegm.

Ginger, Wild

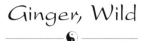

Asarum sieboldii
Xi Xin

Part used: whole Chinese wild ginger plant
Energy and taste: warm; pungent
Affinity: lungs, kidney; treats the exterior
Uses: Wild ginger is used to treat colds; body aches; copious, watery, white phlegm; headaches; toothaches; nasal congestion; and facial nerve pain.
Precautions: Avoid using this herb if yellow phlegm or deficient heat are present.
Dosage: infusion, 1 to 3 grams

Ginseng

Panax ginseng
Ren Shen

Part used: root
Energy and taste: slightly warm; sweet, slightly bitter
Affinity: lungs, spleen; tonifies energy
Uses: Ginseng treats all deficiency diseases with the following symptomology: chronic fatigue; shortness of breath; profuse sweating; lethargy; lack of appetite; chest and abdominal distension; chronic diarrhea; prolapse of the stomach, uterus, or rectum; palpitations accompanied by anxiety; insomnia; forgetfulness; and restlessness. It aids convalescence, and alleviates debility and weakness in the elderly.
Precautions: Do not use ginseng in the presence of deficient heat, excess heat, hypertension, high blood pressure, or when signs of weakness are absent. The consumption of turnips may reduce its effects.
Dosage: decoction, 1 to 9 grams
Note: This herb is Chinese ginseng, which generally consists of the whole root or white powder. When steamed, Chinese ginseng becomes red, and is called Korean ginseng. Korean red ginseng is considered superior in quality.

Green Citrus

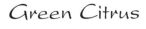

Citrus reticulata
Qing Pi

Part used: green peel of the immature tangerine
Energy and taste: warm; bitter, pungent
Affinity: gallbladder, liver, stomach; regulates energy
Uses: This herb is effective in the treatment of distension; chest, breast, hernial, or side pains; liver, gallbladder, bile, and food congestion; belching; breast abscesses; intermittent fevers and chills; expectoration of lung mucus; and lymphatic congestion. *Qing pi* also raises blood pressure.
Precautions: Avoid use of this herb in the presence of fatigue or weakness.
Dosage: Briefly decoct 3 to 9 grams of *qing pi*.

Gypsum

Calcium sulfate
Shi Gao

Part used: the whole mineral
Energy and taste: very cold; pungent, sweet
Affinity: lungs, stomach; clears heat
Uses: Gypsum is used to relieve a high fever unaccompanied by chills, and for irritability, restlessness, intense thirst, profuse sweating, coughing, expectoration of thick phlegm, headaches, toothaches, and swollen and painful gums.
Precautions: If poor digestion or coldness are present, avoid using gypsum, since it is very cold in energy and hard on the digestion.
Dosage: Decoct 9 to 30 grams of gypsum for 30 minutes, before cooking with other herbs.

Hawthorn

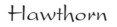

Crataegus spp.
Shan Zha

Part used: fruit
Energy and taste: slightly warm; sour, sweet
Affinity: lungs, spleen, stomach; relieves food stagnation
Uses: *Crataegus* can reduce indigestion, gas, food congestion, abdominal distension, stomach or chest pain, diarrhea, hernia, dysentery, hypertension, coronary-artery disease, and elevated serum cholesterol.
Precautions: Avoid use of this herb in the presence of acid regurgitation or weak digestion unaccompanied by food congestion.
Dosage: decoction, 9 to 15 grams

He Shou Wu

Polygonum multiflorum
He Shou Wu

Part used: root; also known as *ho shou wu* and *fo ti*
Energy and taste: slightly warm; bitter, sweet, astringent
Affinity: liver, kidneys; tonifies blood
Uses: *He shou wu* can treat dizziness; blurred vision; premature graying of hair; premature aging; lower-back pain and weakness; insomnia; nocturnal emissions; spermatorrhea; persistent vaginal discharge; goiters and other neck lumps; carbuncles; sores; constipation resulting from blood deficiency; and chronic malaria accompanied by deficient energy and blood.
Precautions: *He shou wu* should not be used in the presence of weak digestion, phlegm, or diarrhea. Also, this herb should not be consumed with onions, chives, or garlic.
Dosage: Decoct 9 to 30 grams of *he shou wu*. Do not decoct this herb in a steel container, since this preparation adversely alters its properties.

Hoelen

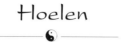

Poria cocos
Fu Ling
(also called tuckahoe and Indian bread)

Part used: sclerotium of the fungus
Energy and taste: neutral; sweet, bland
Affinity: heart, spleen, lungs; diuretic
Uses: Hoelen can alleviate difficult urination, edema, diarrhea, loss of appetite, palpitations, insomnia, and forgetfulness.
Precautions: This herb should not be used in the presence of frequent, cold-induced copious urine. Do not take more than 15 grams of hoelen, or ingest the herb continuously for over a year.
Dosage: decoction, 9 to 15 grams

Honeysuckle

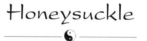

Lonicera japonica
Jin Yin Hua

Part used: flower
Energy and taste: cold; sweet
Affinity: large intestine, lungs, stomach; clears heat and toxins
Uses: Honeysuckle is used to treat acute fevers; sore throats; headaches; dysentery; painful urination; hot, painful sores; and breast, throat, or eye swelling.
Precautions: Do not use this herb in the presence of coldness, poor digestion, or diarrhea.
Dosage: decoction, 9 to 15 grams

Houttuynia

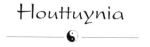

Houttuynia cordata
Yu Xing Cao

Part used: leaves
Energy and taste: cool; pungent
Affinity: large intestine, lungs
Uses: Houttuynia may alleviate pneumonia, bronchitis, or coughing accompanied by thick, yellow-green mucus; abscesses; boils and sores accompanied by pus; and painful urination.
Precautions: Avoid use of this herb if coldness or weakness are present.
Dosage: Decoct 15 to 30 grams of houttuynia for 10 minutes. Use 30 to 60 grams to treat acute conditions.
Note: This herb has a fishy smell.

Isatis

Isatis tinctoria
Ban Lan Gen

Part used: woad root
Energy and taste: cold; bitter
Affinity: heart, lungs, stomach; clears heat and toxins
Uses: Isatis is a broad-spectrum antibiotic. It treats viral infections; fevers; inflammations; mumps; throat pain and swelling; jaundice; acute laryngitis; hepatitis; and scabies.
Precautions: Do not use this herb if weakness is present.
Dosage: decoction, 15 to 30 grams

Jujube Dates

Ziziphus jujuba
Da Zao

Part used: fruit
Energy and taste: neutral; sweet
Affinity: spleen, stomach; tonifies energy
Uses: Jujube dates may alleviate weakness, shortness of breath, lack of appetite, loose stools, and emotional instability. This herb also nourishes blood and *qi*.
Precautions: Avoid use of this herb in the presence of excess heat, food congestion, or intestinal parasites.
Dosage: decoction, 3 to 12 pieces

Leaven, Medicated

Massa fermentata
Shen Qu

Part used: medicated leaven (a non-standard combination of the fermented mixture of wheat, flour, bran, and various other herbs)
Energy and taste: warm; pungent, sweet
Affinity: spleen, stomach; relieves food stagnation
Uses: *Shen qu* regulates food congestion, indigestion, abdominal fullness or distension, lack of appetite, rumbling of the intestines, and diarrhea.
Precautions: Do not use this mixture during pregnancy, while nursing, or in the presence of stomach heat.
Dosage: decoction, 6 to 15 grams

Licorice

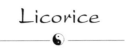

Glycyrrhiza uralensis
Gan Cao

Part used: root
Energy and taste: neutral; sweet
Affinity: Licorice enters all meridians; in particular, it affects the heart, lungs, spleen, and stomach. It also tonifies energy.
Uses: This herb may eliminate shortness of breath; weakness; loose stools; energy or blood deficiencies; palpitations; coughing; wheezing; heat or cold in the lungs; carbuncles; sores; sore throats; painful spasms in the abdomen or legs; and stomach and duodenal ulcers. It also detoxifies poisons. Licorice harmonizes the characteristics of other herbs when added to them, and sweetens a formula.
Precautions: Do not use licorice with polygala, or in the presence of edema accompanied by high blood pressure; a tendency towards fluid retention; nausea; or vomiting.
Dosage: decoction, 2 to 12 grams

Ligusticum

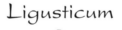

Ligusticum wallichii
Chuan Xiong

Part used: the root of Szechwan lovage, also known as cnidium.
Energy and taste: warm; pungent
Affinity: liver, gallbladder; moves blood
Uses: Ligusticum treats menstrual disorders and pain, including dysmenorrhea and amenorrhea; endometriosis; pain resulting from difficult labor; chest, side, and rib pain and soreness; headaches; dizziness; and skin problems.
Precautions: Ligusticum should not be used with cornus, astragalus, or coptis; or in the presence of deficient heat, weakness, fatigue, or excessive menstrual bleeding. An overdose may result in vomiting and dizziness.
Dosage: decoction, 3 to 9 grams

Ligustrum

☯

Ligustrum lucidum
Nu Zhen Zi

Part used: privet fruit seeds
Energy and taste: neutral; bitter, sweet
Affinity: kidneys, liver; tonifies *yin*
Uses: Ligustrum may alleviate dizziness, the appearance of spots within the field of vision, blurriness of vision, lower-back soreness, premature graying of hair, tinnitus, and deafness.
Precautions: Do not use this herb if poor digestion or diarrhea are present.
Dosage: decoction, 4.5 to 15 grams

Lily Bulb

☯

Lilium brownii
Bai He

Part used: bulb
Energy and taste: slightly cold; sweet, slightly bitter
Affinity: heart, lungs; tonifies *yin*
Uses: This herb treats dry coughing; sore throats; intractable, low-grade fevers; insomnia; restlessness; and palpitations.
Precautions: Avoid use of this herb in the presence of diarrhea or coughing accompanied by white phlegm.
Dosage: decoction, 9 to 30 grams

Lindera

Lindera strychnifolia
Wu Yao

Part used: root
Energy and taste: warm; pungent
Affinity: bladder, kidneys, lungs, spleen; regulates energy
Uses: Lindera alleviates chest, side, and abdominal pain resulting from coldness; stifling sensations in the chest; frequent urination; and urinary incontinence caused by coldness.
Precautions: Avoid use of this herb in the presence of weakness, fatigue, or excess heat.
Dosage: decoction, 3 to 9 grams

Longan Berries

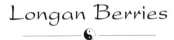

Euphoria longan
Long Yan Rou

Part used: fruit
Energy and taste: warm; sweet
Affinity: heart, spleen; tonifies blood
Uses: Longan berries are used to treat anemia; restlessness; anxiety; palpitations; insomnia; forgetfulness; dizziness; and problems associated with overwork, including stress, fatigue, exhaustion, and palpitations. This herb also has a calming effect.
Dosage: decoction, 6 to 15 grams

Loquat

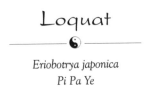

Eriobotrya japonica
Pi Pa Ye

Part used: leaf
Energy and taste: cool; bitter
Affinity: lungs, stomach; stops coughing and wheezing
Uses: Loquat may eliminate coughing accompanied by yellow phlegm, nausea, vomiting caused by heat, hiccups, and belching.
Precautions: Do not use this herb in the presence of cold-induced vomiting.
Dosage: Decoct 4.5 to 12 grams of dry loquat, or 15 to 30 grams of the fresh herb.

Lotus, Seed

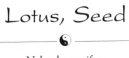

Nelumbo nucifera
Lian Zi

Part used: seeds
Energy and taste: neutral; sweet
Affinity: heart, kidneys, spleen; astringent
Uses: Lotus seed may eliminate chronic diarrhea; loss of appetite; premature ejaculation; spermatorrhea; excessive uterine bleeding; vaginal discharge; palpitations accompanied by anxiety; irritability accompanied by weakness; and insomnia.
Precautions: Avoid use of this herb when abdominal distension or constipation are manifest.
Dosage: decoction, 6 to 15 grams

Lycii Berries

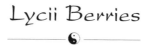

Lycium barbarum
Gou Qi Zi

Part used: Chinese wolfberry fruit
Energy and taste: neutral; sweet
Affinity: liver, lungs, kidneys; tonifies blood
Uses: Lycii berries relieve anemia; dry eyes; dizziness; blurred vision; photosensitivity; night blindness; poor vision; impotence; nocturnal emissions; tuberculosis; and sore backs, knees, and legs.
Precautions: Do not use this herb in the presence of excess heat or loose stools.
Dosage: decoction, 6 to 18 grams

Magnolia, Bark

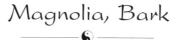

Magnolia officinalis
Hou Po

Part used: bark
Energy and taste: warm; bitter, pungent
Affinity: large intestine, lungs, spleen, stomach; aromatic stomachic
Uses: Magnolia bark treats chronic digestive disturbances accompanied by gas, bloating, colic, chest and abdominal fullness, loss of appetite, vomiting, diarrhea, an acid stomach, expectoration of excess mucus, wheezing, coughing, and lumps in the throat.
Precautions: Magnolia bark should not be used during pregnancy, or with alismatis.
Dosage: decoction, 3 to 9 grams
Note: Magnolia flowers (*Magnolia liliflora* or *xin yi hua*) are also used. It is a specific for nasal congestion, obstruction, or discharge; loss of smell; and sinus problems due to coldness. Infuse 3 to 9 grams of this herb. Avoid use in the presence of *yin*-deficient heat; overuse can cause dizziness or redness of eyes.

Mandarin Orange

Citrus reticulata
Chen Pi

Part used: aged tangerine peel
Energy and taste: warm; pungent, bitter, aromatic
Affinity: lungs, spleen, stomach; regulates energy
Uses: Citrus peel is used to treat indigestion, abdominal distension and fullness, bloating, belching, nausea, vomiting, coughing accompanied by copious phlegm, loss of appetite, fatigue, and loose stools.
Precautions: Avoid use of this herb in the presence of dry coughing, expectoration of yellow phlegm, and expectoration of blood.
Dosage: 10-minute decoction, 3 to 9 grams

Mint

Mentha haplocalyx, M. arvensis
Bo He

Part used: leaves
Energy and taste: cool; pungent
Affinity: lungs, liver; treats the exterior
Uses: Mint may alleviate fevers; headaches; coughing; sore throats; sinus congestion; earaches; the early stages of rashes and skin eruptions, such as measles; reddened eyes and eye inflammations; and indigestion.
Precautions: Avoid use of this herb if severe chills or deficient heat are manifest.
Dosage: infusion, 2 to 6 grams

Morinda

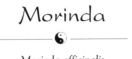

Morinda officinalis
Ba Ji Tian

Part used: root
Energy and taste: warm; pungent, sweet
Affinity: kidneys, liver; tonifies *yang*
Uses: Morinda treats impotence; infertility; premature ejaculation; frequent urination; urinary incontinence; irregular menstruation; cold, painful lower abdomens, backs, and legs; muscular atrophy; bone degeneration; broken bones; and ligament problems. It also strengthens tendons and bones.
Precautions: Morinda should not be used in the presence of deficient heat, difficult urination, or with salvia.
Dosage: decoction, 6 to 15 grams

Morus

Morus alba
Sang Bai Pi

Part used: mulberry-root bark
Energy and taste: cold; sweet
Affinity: lungs, spleen; clears phlegm and stops coughing and wheezing
Uses: Morus alleviates coughing and wheezing accompanied by thick, yellow phlegm; bronchitis; asthma; swelling of the face and extremities; fever; thirst; difficult urination; and hypertension.
Precautions: Avoid use of morus in the presence of excessive urination or coughing accompanied by white phlegm.
Dosage: decoction, 6 to 15 grams

Motherwort

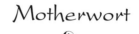

Leonurus heterophyllus
Yi Mu Cao

Part used: parts grown above ground
Energy and taste: slightly cold; pungent, bitter
Affinity: heart, liver, bladder; moves blood
Uses: Motherwort is used to treat menstrual disorders, irregular menstruation, abdominal pain resulting from premenstrual syndrome, abdominal masses, infertility, postpartum abdominal pain, and edema.
Precautions: Do not use motherwort during pregnancy, or in the presence of blood or *yin* deficiencies.
Dosage: infusion, 10 to 30 grams

Mouton

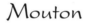

Paeonia suffruticosa
Mu Dan Pi

Part used: cortex of tree peony root
Energy and taste: cool; pungent, bitter
Affinity: heart, liver, kidneys; clears heat, cools blood
Uses: Mouton treats nosebleeds, bloody phlegm or vomit, frequent and profuse menstruation resulting from heat, amenorrhea, dysmenorrhea, abdominal masses, lumps or bruises due to traumatic injury, headaches, and eye pain.
Precautions: Do not use mouton in the presence of coldness or excessive sweating.
Dosage: decoction, 6 to 12 grams

Myrrh

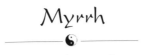

Commiphora myrrha
Mo Yao

Part used: gum resin
Energy and taste: neutral; bitter
Affinity: heart, liver, spleen; moves the blood
Uses: Myrrh alleviates menstrual, chest, abdominal, and trauma-related pain; rheumatism; arthritis; circulatory problems; sores; carbuncles; swellings; immobile abdominal masses; and uterine tumors.
Precautions: This herb must not be used during pregnancy or excessive uterine bleeding.
Dosage: decoction, 3 to 12 grams

Notopterygium

Notopterygium incisum
Qiang Huo

Part used: root
Energy and taste: warm; pungent, bitter
Affinity: bladder, kidney; treats the exterior
Uses: Notopterygium treats chills, fever, flu, headaches, joint pain, and upper-limb and back arthritis pain.
Precautions: Do not use this herb in the presence of weakness, deficient heat, or deficient blood.
Dosage: decoction, 6 to 15 grams

Ophiopogon

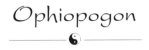

Ophiopogon japonicus
Mai Men Dong

Part used: tuber
Energy and taste: slightly cold; sweet, slightly bitter
Affinity: heart, lungs, stomach; tonifies *yin*
Uses: Ophiopogon relieves dry coughing, expectoration of blood, dryness of the tongue and mouth, irritability, night fever, constipation resulting from dryness, sore throats, and mouth sores.
Precautions: Do not use this herb in the presence of diarrhea resulting from coldness, or with coltsfoot.
Dosage: decoction, 6 to 15 grams

Orzya

Orzya sativa
Gu Ya

Part used: rice sprouts
Energy and taste: neutral; sweet
Affinity: spleen, stomach; relieves food stagnation
Uses: Orzya treats food congestion, poor digestion (especially of starches), loss of appetite, and nausea.
Precautions: Nursing mothers should not use this herb.
Dosage: infusion, 9 to 15 grams

Oyster Shell

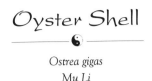

Ostrea gigas
Mu Li

Part used: shell
Energy and taste: cool; salty
Affinity: liver, kidneys; sedative and nervine; astringent
Uses: Oyster shell alleviates palpitations accompanied by anxiety; restlessness; insomnia; irritability; dizziness; headaches; tinnitus; blurred vision; bad temper; spontaneous sweating; night sweats; nocturnal emissions; spermatorrhea; vaginal discharge; uterine bleeding resulting from weakness; heartburn; and neck lumps, such as scrofula and goiter.
Precautions: Do not use this herb in the presence of high fever; or with achyranthes, asarum, ephedra, fritillary, licorice, or polygala. An overdose may lead to indigestion or constipation.
Dosage: Decoct 15 to 30 grams of oyster shell for 60 minutes.

Peony

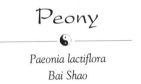

Paeonia lactiflora
Bai Shao

Part used: white-peony root
Energy and taste: cool; bitter, sour
Affinity: liver, spleen; tonifies blood
Uses: Peony regulates menstruation; vaginal discharge; uterine bleeding; anemia; chest, side, or abdominal pain; abdominal spasms; cramps or spasms in hands or feet; headaches; dizziness; spermatorrhea; spontaneous sweating; night sweats; diarrhea; and dysentery.
Precautions: diarrhea resulting from coldness and weakness.
Dosage: decoction, 6 to 15 grams
Note: Wild peony is also used to treat various conditions. Known as red peony, or *chi shao*, it moves blood and helps alleviate abdominal pain, immobile abdominal masses, traumatic injury, dysmenorrhea, and bleeding. Avoid using *chi shao* in the presence of blood deficiency. Decoct 4.5 to 9 grams of this herb.

Perilla

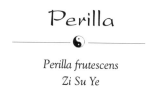

Perilla frutescens
Zi Su Ye

Part used: leaf
Energy and taste: warm; pungent
Affinity: lungs, spleen; treats the exterior
Uses: Perilla effectively treats colds, flu, nasal congestion, coughing, asthma, headaches, nausea, vomiting, abdominal bloating, diarrhea, reduced appetite, restless fetal movement, and morning sickness. It also alleviates seafood poisoning.
Dosage: infusion, 3 to 9 grams

Persica

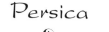

Prunus persica
Tao Ren

Part used: peach kernel
Energy and taste: neutral; bitter, sweet
Affinity: heart, large intestine, liver, lungs; moves blood
Uses: Persica may relieve menstrual disorders, delayed menses, tumors, abdominal pain, pain resulting from traumatic injuries, side pain, lungs and intestinal abscesses, immobile abdominal masses, and constipation resulting from dryness.
Precautions: Do not use this herb during pregnancy.
Dosage: decoction, 4.5 to 9 grams

Phellodendron

— ☯ —

Phellodendron amurense
Huang Bai

Part used: amur cork-tree bark
Energy and taste: cold; bitter
Affinity: kidneys, bladder; clears damp heat
Uses: Phellodendron alleviates thick, yellow vaginal discharge; gonorrhea; foul-smelling diarrhea; dysentery; red, swollen, and painful knees, legs, or feet; jaundice; night sweats; nocturnal emissions; spermatorrhea; and mouth or gum sores.
Precautions: Do not use this herb when weak digestion is present.
Dosage: decoction, 3 to 12 grams

Pinellia

— ☯ —

Pinellia ternata
Ban Xia

Part used: rhizome
Energy and taste: warm; pungent; toxic
Affinity: lungs, spleen, stomach; clears phlegm and cold
Uses: Pinella alleviates coughing or bronchitis characterized by copious white phlegm; bronchial congestion; vomiting; nausea; weak digestion; abdominal distention; and nodules, especially in the neck.
Precautions: Use prepared pinellia—deep-fried with ginger, vinegar, or alumen—exclusively. Do not use pinellia when bleeding or deficient heat are present, or with aconite.
Dosage: decoction, 4 to 12 grams

Platycodon

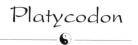

Platycodon grandiflorum
Jie Geng

Part used: balloon-flower root
Energy and taste: neutral; bitter, pungent
Affinity: lungs; clears phlegm and stops coughing
Uses: Platycodon is used to eliminate coughing and phlegm, in both hot and cold conditions; sore throats; loss of voice; lung or throat abscesses; and pus in the upper parts of body.
Precautions: Do not use this herb in the presence of blood expectoration, or with gentian.
Dosage: decoction, 3 to 9 grams

Polygala

Polygala tenufolia
Yuan Zhi

Part used: Chinese senega root
Energy and taste: slightly warm; bitter, pungent
Affinity: heart, lungs; calmative
Uses: Polygala may alleviate anxious palpitations, insomnia, restlessness, poor memory, mental and emotional disorientation, pent-up emotions, seizures, coughing accompanied by copious mucus, boils, abscesses, sores, and swollen and painful breasts.
Precautions: Avoid use of polygala in the presence of deficient heat, ulcers, or gastritis.
Dosage: decoction, 3 to 9 grams

Polygonati

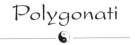

Polygonatum sibiricum
Huang Jing

Part used: Siberian Solomon's seal rhizome
Energy and taste: neutral; sweet
Affinity: kidneys, lungs, spleen; tonifies energy
Uses: Polygonati is used to treat fatigue, a dry mouth, loss of appetite, dry stools, dry coughing, lower-back pain, lightheadedness, weak legs, and thirst.
Precautions: Avoid use of this herb when poor digestion is manifest.
Dosage: Decoct 6 to 18 grams of this herb. Polygonati can be used as a long-term treatment.

Polyporus

Polyporus umbellatus
Zhu Ling

Part used: polyporus sclerotium
Energy and taste: slightly cool; sweet
Affinity: spleen, kidney, bladder; diuretic
Uses: Polyporus treats difficult urination; cloudy, painful urination; kidney stones; nephritis; edema; vaginal discharge; diarrhea; and jaundice.
Precautions: Long-term use of this herb can cause deficient heat.
Dosage: decoction, 6 to 15 grams

Pseudoginseng

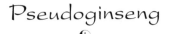

Panax notoginseng, P. pseudoginseng
San Qi
(also known as Tien Qi ginseng)

Part used: root
Energy and taste: warm; sweet, slightly bitter
Affinity: liver, stomach, large intestine; regulates blood
Uses: Pseudoginseng treats internal and external bleeding, vomiting, nose-bleeds, bloody urine or stools, fractures, contusions, sprains, chest and abdominal pain, and menstrual pain.
Precautions: Do not use this herb during pregnancy, or in the presence of blood or *yin* deficiencies.
Dosage: decoction, 3 to 9 grams; powder, 1 to 3 grams

Psoralea

Psoralea corylifolia
Bu Gu Zhi

Part used: seeds
Energy and taste: very warm; pungent, bitter
Affinity: kidneys, spleen; tonifies *yang*
Uses: Psoralea may eliminate impotence; premature ejaculation; leukorrhea; lower-back pain, coldness, and weakness; urinary incontinence; frequent urination; spermatorrhea; diarrhea; rumbling of the intestines; abdominal pain; wheezing; baldness; and psoriasis. This herb also has antifungal properties.
Precautions: Do not use this herb with licorice, or in the presence of deficient heat, constipation, or poor digestion.
Dosage: Crush 3 to 9 grams of psoralea, then decoct.

Pueraria

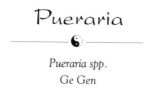

Pueraria spp.
Ge Gen

Part used: kudzu-vine root
Energy and taste: cool; pungent, sweet
Affinity: spleen, stomach; treats the exterior
Uses: Pueraria treats fevers, headaches, a tight neck and shoulders, dizziness, thirst, dehydration, hypertension, chronic diarrhea, measles, and other skin eruptions.
Dosage: decoction, 6 to 12 grams
Note: the flowers are used for alcohol and drug poisoning.

Radish

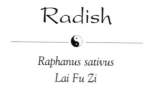

Raphanus sativus
Lai Fu Zi

Part used: seeds
Energy and taste: neutral; pungent, sweet
Affinity: lungs, spleen, stomach; relieves food stagnation
Uses: Radish seed is used to alleviate food congestion, indigestion, abdominal fullness and distension, belching accompanied by a rotten smell, acid regurgitation, abdominal pain accompanied by diarrhea, coughing accompanied by phlegm, and wheezing.
Precautions: Do not use this herb in the presence of weakness or fatigue.
Dosage: decoction, 6 to 12 grams

Rehmannia, Cooked

— ☯ —

Rehmannia glutinosa
Shu Di Huang

Part used: Chinese foxglove root, cooked in wine
Energy and taste: slightly warm; sweet
Affinity: heart, kidneys, liver; tonifies blood
Uses: Rehmannia may eliminate anemia; dizziness; blurred vision; palpitations; insomnia; irregular menstruation; uterine and postpartum bleeding, caused by weakness; night sweats; nocturnal emissions; lower-back pain; weakness of the legs; lightheadedness; tinnitus; infertility; impotence; loss of hearing; and premature graying of hair.
Precautions: Overuse of this herb can lead to abdominal distension and loose stools.
Dosage: decoction, 9 to 30 grams
Note: Uncooked rehmannia, called *sheng di huang*, is also used. It has a cold energy, and is a specific for very high fevers; continuous, low-grade fevers; thirst; dryness of the mouth; constipation; mouth and tongue sores; irritability; insomnia; malar flush; nosebleeds; bloody phlegm, vomit, or urine; and uterine bleeding. Do not use this herb in the presence of diarrhea, coldness, or anemia. Decoct 9 to 30 grams of *sheng di huang*.

Reishi

— ☯ —

Ganoderma spp. (especially lucidum)
Ling Zhi
(also called ganoderma)

Part used: whole mushroom
Energy and taste: neutral; bitter
Affinity: heart, liver, lungs, entire body; tonifies energy, sedative
Uses: Reishi is used to treat fatigue, AIDS, cancer, tumors, heart disease, cholesterol, high blood pressure, allergies, bronchitis, asthma, pneumonia, rheumatism, insomnia, dizziness, hepatitis, stress, liver diseases, fatigue, and lack of strength.
Dosage: Decoct 3 to 15 grams of *ling zhi* for 1 hour.

Rhubarb

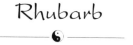

Rheum palmatum
Da Huang

Part used: root and rhizome
Energy and taste: cold; bitter
Affinity: large intestine, liver, stomach; purgative
Uses: Rhubarb may alleviate constipation, high fever, profuse sweating, abdominal distension and pain, delirium, jaundice, dysentery, painful urination, bleeding hemorrhoids, vomiting of blood, nosebleeds accompanied by constipation, abdominal masses, swollen and painful eyes, and hot skin lesions.
Precautions: *Da huang* should not be used during pregnancy or menstruation; in the presence of *qi* or blood deficiencies, coldness, or diarrhea; or by postpartum or nursing mothers.
Dosage: Decoct 3 to 12 grams of the herb; cooking rhubarb for longer than 10 minutes reduces its purgative effect.

Salvia

Salvia miltiorrhiza
Dan Shen

Part used: root
Energy and taste: slightly cold; bitter
Affinity: heart, liver; moves blood
Uses: Salvia relieves painful menstruation, amenorrhea, endometriosis, abdominal masses and pain, chest pain, sore ribs, irritability, palpitations, and insomnia.
Dosage: decoction, 6 to 15 grams

Saussurea

Aucklandia lappa
Mu Xiang

Part used: root
Energy and taste: warm; pungent, bitter
Affinity: gallbladder, large intestine, spleen, stomach; regulates energy
Uses: Saussurea is used to treat lack of appetite, abdominal or chest pain and distension, nausea, and vomiting.
Precautions: deficient heat or dryness
Dosage: Decoct 1.5 to 9 grams of saussurea for 5 minutes.

Scallion

Allium pstulosum
Cong Bai

Part used: white part
Energy and taste: warm; pungent
Affinity: lungs, stomach; treats the exterior
Uses: Scallion effectively treats the early stages of colds and fevers, and sensations of coldness. It also induces sweating, and is a topical treatment for skin sores and abscesses.
Precautions: Do not use this herb in the presence of profuse sweating.
Dosage: infusion, two to five scallions

Schisandra

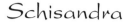

Schisandra chinensis
Wu Wei Zi

Part used: seed
Energy and taste: warm; sour
Affinity: heart, kidneys, lungs; astringent
Uses: Schisandra is used to treat chronic coughing, wheezing resulting from weakness, diarrhea, nocturnal emissions, spermatorrhea, vaginal discharge, frequent urination, excessive sweating, night sweats, irritability, palpitations, insomnia, and dream-disturbed sleep.
Precautions: Do not use this herb in the presence of colds, flu, fevers, or the early stages of rashes or coughs. Schisandra may cause heartburn.
Dosage: decoction, 1.5 to 9 grams

Schizonepeta

Schizonepeta tenuifolia
Jing Jie

Part used: parts grown above ground
Energy and taste: slightly warm; pungent
Affinity: lungs, liver; treats the exterior
Uses: Schizonepeta may alleviate colds, flu, headaches, skin eruptions, and sore throats. When directly applied, fried schizonepeta stops bleeding.
Precautions: Do not use this herb in the presence of fully erupted skin lesions, such as measles.
Dosage: infusion, 3 to 9 grams

Scute

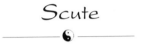

Scutellaria baicalensis
Huang Qin

Part used: baical skullcap root
Energy and taste: cold; bitter
Affinity: gallbladder, large intestine, lungs, stomach; clears damp heat
Uses: Scute treats high fever; irritability; thirst; coughing accompanied by thick, yellow mucus; hot sores and swellings; jaundice; vomiting or expectoration of blood; nosebleeds; bloody stools; reddened eyes; a flushed face; and hypertension.
Precautions: Do not use this herb in the presence of deficient lung heat, coldness, or with mouton.
Dosage: decoction, 6 to 15 grams

Siler

Ledebouriella divaricata
Fang Feng

Part used: root
Energy and taste: slightly warm; pungent, sweet
Affinity: bladder, liver, spleen; treats the exterior
Uses: Siler alleviates migraine headaches, chills, body aches, trembling of the hands and feet, and tetany.
Precautions: Do not use this herb in the presence of anemia or deficient heat, or with ginger.
Dosage: decoction, 3 to 9 grams

Stephania

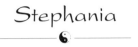

Stephania tetrandra
Han Fang Ji

Part used: root
Energy and taste: cold; bitter, pungent
Affinity: bladder, spleen, kidneys; diuretic
Uses: This herb is used to treat edema; difficult urination; swollen legs; abdominal distension; intestinal gurgling; red, swollen, hot, and painful joints; and knee inflammation.
Precautions: Avoid use of this herb in the presence of deficient heat.
Dosage: decoction, 3 to 9 grams

Tribulus

Tribulus terrestris
Bai Ji Li

Part used: fruit
Energy and taste: warm; bitter, pungent
Affinity: liver, lungs; extinguishes wind, stops spasms
Uses: Tribulus treats headaches; dizziness; red, swollen, and painful eyes; insufficient lactation; chest or side pain; itching; hives; and increases the eyes' ability to tear.
Precautions: Tribulus should not be used during pregnancy, or when blood or energy deficiencies are present.
Dosage: decoction, 6 to 12 grams

Trichosanthes

Trichosanthes kirilowii
Tian Hua Fen

Part used: root
Energy and taste: cold; bitter, slightly sweet
Affinity: lungs, stomach; clears phlegm and stops coughing
Uses: Trichosanthes treats tuberculosis, dry coughing, blood-streaked sputum, thirst, irritability, abscesses, swellings, and tumors.
Precautions: Avoid use of this herb during pregnancy, or when coldness, diarrhea, pregnancy, and poor digestion are present.
Dosage: decoction, 9 to 15 grams

Wormwood

Artemisia annua
Qing Hao

Part used: Chinese wormwood leaves
Energy and taste: cold; bitter
Affinity: kidney, liver, gallbladder; treats the exterior
Uses: Wormword treats fevers accompanied by weakness; night fevers characterized by morning coolness and lack of sweat; alternating fever and chills; malaria; nosebleeds; summer flu accompanied by low fevers; headaches; dizziness; and a stuffy sensation in the chest.
Precautions: Postpartum women with deficient blood or individuals with weak digestion should not use this herb. Do not use wormwood with rehmannia or *dang gui*.
Dosage: Decoct 3 to 9 grams of this herb for a maximum of 10 minutes.
Note: The Red Cross uses this herb to treat malaria.

Yam, Wild

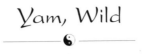

Dioscorea opposita
Shan Yao

Part used: Chinese wild-yam root
Energy and taste: neutral; sweet
Affinity: kidneys, lungs, spleen; tonifies energy
Uses: Chinese wild yam regulates diarrhea, fatigue, spontaneous sweating, lack of appetite, chronic coughing or wheezing caused by weak lungs, spermatorrhea, frequent urination, vaginal discharge, and diabetes.
Precautions: Do not use this herb if excess heat or congestion are present.
Dosage: decoction, 9 to 30 grams

Zanthoxylum

Zanthoxylum bungeanum
Chuan Jiao

Part used: Szechwan pepper fruit and Chinese prickly ash
Energy and taste: hot; pungent, slightly toxic
Affinity: kidneys, spleen, stomach; warms interior
Uses: Zanthoxylum alleviates abdominal pain and coldness, vomiting, diarrhea, intestinal parasites, and pain caused by roundworms.
Precautions: Do not use this herb in the presence of deficient heat, or with coltsfoot.
Dosage: Decoct 1.5 to 6 grams of zanthoxylum for 5 minutes. This herb can also be used externally, as a compress applied directly over the painful area.

Zizyphus

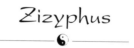

Zizyphus spinosa
Suan Zao Ren

Part used: sour jujube seed

Energy and taste: neutral; sweet, sour

Affinity: gallbladder, heart, liver, spleen; calmative

Uses: Zizyphus is used to treat insomnia, palpitations accompanied by anxiety, irritability, spontaneous sweating, night sweats, forgetfulness, and nervous exhaustion.

Precautions: Avoid use of this herb in the presence of severe diarrhea or excess heat.

Dosage: Crush 9 to 18 grams of zizyphus, then decoct the herb.

Chinese Herbal Patent Medicines

Chinese patents are herbal formulas in convenient forms, including pills, syrups, powders, and liniments. Patents are effective, economical, easy to carry, can be stored for long periods of time, and (generally speaking) have an innocuous taste. These treatments were first used over 2,000 years ago, and they have proven themselves in clinical application.

When taken properly, most patents offer significant benefits without side effects. Many patents are quite effective in the treatment of acute conditions such as colds, flu, fevers, trauma, and pain. The convenience of patents also makes them the best therapy for chronic conditions.

The creation of Chinese patents: Chinese patents are carefully grown, harvested, and processed in China. Entire villages work together to cultivate the plants used in patents. Many highly respected North American practitioners have viewed the patent production process, and can attest to its quality. Most patents are made by boiling herbs down in a tea and drying the resulting mass. Pills are often sugarcoated, to preserve them and prevent them from melting together.

How to take patents: Patents are best taken 30 minutes before or after meals, with room-temperature or warm water or tea. They are best absorbed when chewed, if taste permits. Certain foods must be avoided in conjunction with certain patents; for example, beans and seafood should not be consumed when an individual is taking patents for arthritis and rheumatism.

Chinese patents are generally packaged in corked glass bottles and topped by plastic twist caps. Use a small knife to remove the cork; carefully ease the knife, at an angle, into the side of the cork and gently pull it out. Corkscrews are also effective. Other patents—in the form of large, soft balls—are contained by wax "eggs." Press the egg to pop it open. The patent-medicine balls are chewed or cut into smaller pieces and swallowed.

Patents may be taken alone or in combination. Medicines taken together enhance one another's effects. A cold and cough may be treated with *Ganmaoling* and a syrup, such as *Hsiao Keh Chuan*. Irregular periods, premenstrual syndrome, poor digestion, lung phlegm, and abdominal fullness are regulated by *Hsiao Yao Wan* and *Erh Chen Wan*.

Duration of patent treatment: Most patents are taken until the targeted symptoms subside. Tonics that increase energy or build blood and patents used to treat chronic conditions are the exceptions to this rule. Their effectiveness should be evaluated periodically.

Dosages: In the treatment of acute cases for short periods, or to achieve quicker results, it is fairly common to increase dosages by 50 to 100 percent. Give up to twice the recommended dosage of principal-therapy patents for a few days to a week, and then return to the indicated dosage. Pediatric dosages are reduced according to age, as follows: 0 to 3 years, less than one-third dose; 3 to 7 years, one-third dosage; 7 to 15 years, one-half dosage; over 15 years, adult dosage.

Cautions: Patents with important contraindications or cautions are listed here. Pregnancy is the most common contraindication. Some formulas, when improperly used, may impair digestion or cause diarrhea. It is critical to heed these cautions.

Obtaining patents: Patents may be obtained from Chinese pharmacies in the Chinatowns of major cities, in health-food stores, from acupuncture practitioners, and from Chinese herbal-patent distributors. Many suppliers sell by mail order; some of these suppliers are listed in the "Recommended Reading and Sources" appendix, on page 188.

Animal products: Several patents contain animal products, because of the potent effects of these products. Animal-product constituents contain substances quite similar to those found in human bodies. Examples of animal products include: rhinoceros horn, antelope horn, gecko lizard, deer antler, pig placenta, tiger bone, and oyster shell. Vegetarians may object to the inclusion of these products; usually, it's possible to find substitute patents. Rhinoceros horn and tiger bone are restricted in North America. As such, patents containing either of these products are not listed below.

Western drugs in Chinese patents: In general, the Chinese do not mix Western drugs into Chinese herbal patents. Patents known to include Western drugs are not listed below.

Note: The patents listed below are generally safe and do not produce side effects. These formulas are only a few of the hundreds available; a visit to a Chinese pharmacy can be eye-opening. It is always wise to seek the advice of a professional when seeking the appropriate patents for treatment of your condition.

To help identify patent forms, use the following guidelines: "*wan*" is a round pill, "*san*" is a powder, "*gao*" is a plaster, and "*dan*" is a patent medicine that contains minerals.

Chinese herbal patents can be divided into the categories listed below. These categories are not traditional classifications; they are given to facilitate easy reference and use. Some of the most common patents are not listed below, since they contain prohibited substances such as tiger bone. Most patents containing animal products are not listed. For a clarification of different uses of patents in each category, refer to the chapter entitled "Simple Remedies for Common Ailments," on page 150.

Patent Categories

- colds and flu
- coughing, phlegm, and labored breathing
- headaches

- allergies and sinus infections
- sore throats, mouth disorders, and ear problems
- eye disorders
- genitourinary conditions
- hemorrhoids
- gynecological conditions
- digestive disorders
- liver and gallbladder disorders
- heart disorders
- skin disorders
- arthritis and rheumatism
- restlessness and insomnia
- hypertension
- energy tonics
- pediatric disorders
- pain
- trauma

Colds and Flu

Ganmaoling tablets

Ganmaoling is one of the most commonly known and used Chinese herbal patents; it is an excellent treatment for colds and flu accompanied by chills; high fever; swollen lymph glands; sore throats; and upper-back and neck stiffness. If taken prior to the onset of cold or flu, it may also prevent these illnesses.

Dose: *Ganmaoling* is available in 36-tablet bottles. To prevent colds, take two tablets two to three times a day for three days. During the acute stages of a cold, take three to six tablets three times a day.

Yin Chiao Tablets (Tianjin)

There are several types of *Yin Chiao* Tablets. Superior Quality—Sugar Coated, which is a particular brand of *Yin Chiao*, includes antelope horn and Western chemicals. Do not use this brand. Other brands are effective; they differ from one another only in the amount of herb content. The *Tianjin* brand contains more herbs.

Like *Ganmaoling, Yin Chiao* is commonly used in the treatment of flu, colds, measles, tonsillitis, pneumonia, swollen lymph nodes, sore throats, body aches, fevers accompanied by chills, headaches, thirst, sore shoulders, stiff necks, itching skin accompanied by an aversion to heat, and hives. This compound promotes sweating.

Dose: Yin Chiao can be purchased in boxes containing 12 bottles; each bottle holds eight pills. One-hundred-pill bottles are also available. Take five to six pills every two to three hours during the first nine hours of illness. After the first nine hours, take five to six pills every four to five hours, as needed. Discontinue use of this patent by the third day of illness.

Zhong Gan Ling

This remedy (similar to *Ganmaoling* tablets) is indicated for stronger heat conditions such as severe colds; flu; sudden, high fevers accompanied by sore throats; swollen lymph nodes; aching limbs; headaches; coughing; and slight chills. This patent promotes sweating.

Caution: Do not use *Zhong Gan Ling* in the presence of strong chills.

Dose: Zhong Gan Ling can be purchased in 48-tablet bottles. Take four to six tablets three to four times a day.

Huo Hsiang Cheng Chi Pien

Also known as Lopanthus Antifebrile Pills, this patent is an effective regulator of colds and flu accompanied by diarrhea; vomiting; abdominal pain accompanied by gurgling and gas; nausea; fever; chills; and headaches. It may also be taken as a treatment for weak digestion characterized by loose stools, or by pregnant women to alleviate morning sickness.

Caution: Do not use this patent in the presence of dry mouth, thirst, and fever without chills.

Dose: This patent is available in 100-pill bottles, or vials containing 12 tablets. Take 10 pills, or four to eight tablets, three times a day.

Chuan Xiong Chao Tiao Wan

This patent treats sudden headaches resulting from a cold accompanied by chills; nasal congestion; sinusitis; and rhinitis.

Dose: Chuan Xiong Chao Tiao Wan can be purchased in 200-pill bottles. Take eight pills three to five times a day.

See the following pages for treatment of:

Stomach flu accompanied by sudden and violent abdominal cramping; bloating accompanied by pain; vomiting; headaches; constipation; or diarrhea. Refer to **Pill Curing** under "Digestive Disorders," on page 116.

Coughing, Phlegm, and Labored Breathing

Bronchitis Pills (Compound)

These pills are useful in the regulation of acute and chronic bronchitis, chronic asthma, and coughing and phlegm caused by colds and flu. Bronchitis Pills also resolve labored breathing resulting from weak lungs and phlegm retention.

Dose: Bronchitis Pills are available in 60-capsule bottles. Take two to three capsules three times a day.

Ching Fei Yi Huo Pian

This herbal patent is used to treat toxic heat accompanied by profuse or sticky, yellow phlegm; dry or raspy coughing; swollen and painful throats; fevers; dark-yellow and scant urine; constipation; mouth or nose sores; bleeding gums; and toothaches.

Dose: Ching Fei Yi Huo Pian can be obtained in boxes containing 12 tubes; each tube holds eight tablets. Take four tablets two to three times a day.

Caution: Discontinue use of this patent after heat symptoms subside or if diarrhea develops. Ingestion of Ching Fei Yi Huo Pian during pregnancy is prohibited.

Pulmonary Tonic Pills

These pills strengthen lungs against chronic lung-weakness symptoms accompanied by heat; these symptoms include dry coughing and the expectoration of sticky, yellow phlegm.

Dose: Pulmonary Tonic Pills are available in 60-pill bottles. Take five pills three times a day.

Erh Chen Wan

This formula is primary in dissolving stomach, lung, or face phlegm congestion accompanied by nausea; abdominal distension; chest distension; dizziness; vertigo; lung phlegm; postnasal drip; nasal mucus; throat phlegm; excessive salivation; and an alcohol-induced hangover.

Dose: Erh Chen Wan is available in 200-pill bottles. Take eight pills three times a day.

Ping Chuan pills

This patent remedies chronic asthma, bronchitis, emphysema, coughing, and shortness of breath that is worse in the evening, all of which are aggravated by overexertion accompanied by lower-back pain; frequent nighttime urination; and weakness. *Ping Chuan* Pills contain gecko lizard, which is an animal product.

Dose: Ping Chuan is available in 120-pill bottles. Take 10 pills three times a day.

Hsiao Keh Chuan pills

Hsiao keh chuan pills are an excellent remedy for acute or chronic bronchitis and asthma; coughing accompanied by copious, clear-to-white mucus; coldness; lung congestion; and difficult breathing.

Dose: These pills can be purchased in 18-capsule bottles. Take two capsules three times a day.

Pinellia Expectorant Pills (Qing Qi Hua Tan Wan)

These pills regulate lung, throat, and sinus heat and mucus; bronchial congestion; sinus congestion; and asthma accompanied by excessive, yellow, thick, sticky phlegm or nasal discharge.

Dose: Pinellia Expectorant Pills are available in 200-pill bottles. Take six pills three times a day.

Caution: Do not use this patent in the presence of chills or dry coughing without phlegm.

See the following pages for treatment of:

Coughing and nasal congestion. Refer to **Bi Yan Pian** under "Allergies and Sinus Infections," on page 107.

Coughing and poor digestion, poor appetite, loose stools, or diarrhea. Refer to **Liu Jun Zi Tablets** under "Digestive Disorders," on page 115.

Hsiao Keh Chuan (Special Bronchitis Medicine)

This fluid regulates acute or chronic bronchitis; coughing accompanied by clear-to-white, watery phlegm; asthma; coldness; and lung weakness, all of which are accompanied by lower-back pain. It also alleviates frequent, clear urination and increases the body's resistance to disease.

Dose: This patent is available in 100-milliliter bottles. Take one to two tablespoons three times a day, alone or with warm water.

Lo Han Kuo tea

Lo Han Kuo treats coughing accompanied by sticky or bloody phlegm; thirst; itchy throats; and chronic coughing, often associated with whooping cough or tuberculosis. This tea is pleasant tasting and easy to prepare.

Dose: One large box contains 12 small boxes of this tea; each small box includes two cubes of the herb. Dissolve one cube in one cup of hot water, and consume this dosage three to six times per day.

Natural Herb Loquat-Flavored Syrup

Use this syrup to treat acute and chronic coughing caused by lung weakness, heat, or dryness accompanied by sticky phlegm. Loquat-flavored syrup also regulates emphysema, acute bronchitis, and accompanying sinus congestion.

Dose: This syrup is available in 5-ounce, 10-ounce, and 15-ounce bottles. Adults should take one tablespoon three times a day; children should ingest one teaspoon three times a day.

Headaches

See the following pages for treatment of:

Headaches and fever. Refer to **Yin Chiao** Tablets or **Zhong Gan Ling** under "Colds and Flu," on page 102.

Headaches and allergies or sinusitis. Refer to **Bi Yan Pian** under "Allergies and Sinus Infections," on page 107.

Headaches and indigestion. Refer to **Pill Curing** under "Digestive Disorders," on page 116.

Headaches and muscle tension or spasms. Refer to **Hsiao Yao Wan** under "Gynecological Conditions," on page 112.

Migraine pain. Refer to **Corydalis Yanhusus Analgesic Tablets** under

"Pain," on page 127.

Migraine pain and sensations of coldness. Refer to **Tian Ma Wan** under "Arthritis and Rheumatism," on page 121.

Headaches and chills. Refer to **Chuan Xiong Chao Tiao Wan** under "Colds and Flu," on page 103.

Allergies and Sinus Infections

Bi Yan Pian

This patent treats sneezing, itchy eyes; facial congestion; and sinus pain. It is also useful in the regulation of acute or chronic rhinitis; sinusitis; hay fever; nasal allergies; stuffy nose; yellowish, thick, foul-smelling sinus discharge; and facial, mucosal congestion.

Dose: Bi Yan Pian is available in 100-bottle tablets. Take four to six tablets three to five times daily.

Pe Min Kan Wan

Pe Min Kan Wan alleviates hay fever; sinus infections; rhinitis; acute or chronic sinusitis; and facial congestion accompanied by sneezing, a runny nose, itchy, watery eyes, and postnasal drip. This patent is a specific for postnasal drip.

Dose: Pe Min Kan Wan can be purchased in 50-pill bottles. Take three pills three times a day.

See the following pages for treatment of:

Sinus congestion and thick, sticky, yellow mucus. Refer to **Pinellia Expectorant Pills (Qing Qi Hua Tan Wan)** under "Coughing, Phlegm, and Labored Breathing," on page 105.

Headaches and sinusitis, rhinitis, nasal congestion, and coldness. Refer to **Chuan Xiong Chao Tiao Wan** under "Colds and Flu," on page 103.

Sore Throats, Mouth Disorders, and Ear Problems

Huang Lien Shang Ching Pien

This patent regulates heat conditions, including high fever; headaches; sore throats; ear infections; itching; hives; swollen gums; toothaches; nosebleeds; insomnia; reddened eyes; constipation; diarrhea; and concentrated, scant urine.

Dose: This treatment is available in boxes containing 12 tubes (with 8 tablets per tube) or in 20-tablet bottles. Take four tablets one to two times a day.

Caution: Stop taking this medication when the above-named heat symptoms subside. Discontinue use of this product if frequent, loose stools develop. Use of this treatment during pregnancy is prohibited.

Chuan Xin Lian (Antiphlogistic Pills)

These pills regulate acute throat inflammations (such as strep) accompanied by swollen glands and fever. *Chuan Xin Lian* alleviates viral infections that cause fever, such as the measles, flu, and hepatitis. It is also used to treat furuncles, mastitis, and abscesses.

Dose: Chuan Xin Lian can be purchased in 60-pill bottles. Take three pills three times a day, for one to four days.

Laryngitis Pills

These pills relieve laryngitis caused by heat. It is also used to treat acute tonsillitis; acute mumps; and hot, lingering sore throats. If these symptoms include a strep infection, take a combination of Laryngitis Pills and *Chuan Xin Lian* (Antiphlogistic Pills). Laryngitis Pills contain animal products.

Dose: These pills come in small boxes, each of which contains three vials; each vial holds 10 pills. Take this medication three times a day, as follows: 0 to 1 year, take 1 pill; 1 to 2 years, take 2 pills; 2 to 3 years, take 3 to 4 pills; 4 to 8 years, take 5 to 6 pills; 9 to 15 years, take 8 to 9 pills. Adults should take 10 pills.

Caution: Restrict ingestion of this patent to a short period of time, one to three days at most. Use of this treatment during pregnancy is prohibited.

Xi Gua Shuang

This watermelon "frost" effectively heals mouth sores, mouth ulcers, and toothaches. It also treats skin burns.

Dose: Xi Gua Shuang comes in boxes, each of which contains 10 vials; each vial holds 2 grams of powder. Mix 1 to 2 grams of powder with water; ingest this mixture two to three times a day. To treat the skin, mix two vials of powder with cooking oil; apply this mixture topically until the burn is healed.

Caution: Do not eat greasy, oily food over the course of this treatment.

Superior Sore Throat Powder Spray

This spray is used to alleviate sore throats; mouth ulcers; ulcerative skin lesions; inflamed sinuses; and hot, middle-ear infections. Superior Sore Throat Powder Spray is effective but bad tasting.

Dose: This powder spray comes in 2.2-gram bottles. To treat: the throat and mouth, spray once, three times a day; sinusitis, spray in the nose, five times a day; oozing middle-ear inflammations, wash with hydrogen peroxide and spray once daily; ulcerative skin lesions, spray once daily.

Tso-Tzu Otic Pills

These pills treat tinnitus (ear ringing), headaches, insomnia, thirst, eye irritation, pressure behind the eyes, and high blood pressure.

Dose: Tso-Tzu Otic Pills are available in 200-pill bottles. Take eight pills three times a day.

See the following pages for treatment of:

Painful and swollen sore throats, nose sores, mouth sores, toothaches, nosebleeds, and swollen gums. Refer to **Ching Fei Yi Huo Pian** under "Coughing, Phlegm, and Labored Breathing," on page 104.

Sore throats; fever blisters; red, burning eyes; headaches; scant urine; and constipation. Refer to **Lung Tan Xie Gan Pills** under "Genitourinary Conditions," on page 111.

Eye Disorders

Ming Mu Shang Ching Pien

This patent alleviates red, itching, and tearing eyes; swelling of the eyes (conjunctivitis); vertigo; photophobia; night blindness; scant, dark urine; constipation; night sweats; fatigue; dry throats; dry mouths; and fever.

Dose: Ming Mu Shang Ching Pien is available in boxes (each of which holds 12 vials; vials contain eight tablets) or in 200-pill bottles. Take 4 tablets two times a day, or 10 pills three times a day.

Caution: Use of this patent during pregnancy is prohibited.

Dendrobium Moniliforme Night Sight Pills

Dendrobium Moniliforme Night Sight Pills treat diminished vision (especially diminished sight accompanied by blurriness); photophobia; cataracts; eye tearing; red, itchy, or dry eyes; hypertensive pressure behind the eyes; night sweats; fatigue; lower-back pain; and insomnia. This patent contains some animal products.

Dose: These pills come in boxes containing 10 pills; each pill holds 6 grams. They are also available in honey-pill form. Take one pill two times a day, or one honey pill two times a day.

See the following pages for treatment of:

Red, burning eyes; sore throats; fever blisters in the mouth; headaches; scant urine; or constipation. Refer to **Lung Tan Xie Gan Pills** under "Genitourinary Conditions," on page 111.

Genitourinary Conditions

Chien Chin Chih Tai Wan

This patent effectively relieves leukorrhea accompanied by white discharge; trichomonas; vaginal infections accompanied by anemia; and vaginal infections accompanied by weaknesses, such as lower-back pain, fatigue, abdominal distension, and abdominal pain.

Dose: Chien Chin Chih Tai Wan can be purchased in 120-pill bottles. Take 10 pills one to two times a day.

Yudai Wan

Yudai Wan treats dark and odorous leukorrhea; and acute vaginitis accompanied by lower-back pain, fatigue, abdominal distension, and abdominal pain. This patent also alleviates bladder infections caused by yeast.

Dose: Yudai Wan can be purchased in 100-pill bottles. Take eight pills three times a day.

Lung Tan Xie Gan Pills

These pills effectively relieve urinary bladder infections; oral herpes; genital herpes; prostatitis; urethritis; red, burning eyes; sore throats; fever blisters in the mouth; scant urine; constipation; and leukorrhea accompanied by yellow discharge.

Dose: This patent is available in 100-pill bottles. Take six pills two times a day.

Eight-Flavor Tea (Chih Pai Di Huang Wan)

Eight-Flavor Tea alleviates bladder or vaginal infections accompanied by a dry throat, thirst, hot flashes, night sweats, hot feet or palms, insomnia, and restless sleep.

Dose: This patent is available in 200-pill bottles. Take eight to sixteen pills three times a day.

Specific Drug Passwan

Passwan treats acute or chronic urinary calculi (stones) in the kidney, bladder, and ureters. It dissolves calculi, and stops bleeding and pain.

Dose: This patent is available in 120-capsule bottles. Take six to eight capsules three times a day.

Kai Kit Wan

This patent is a specific remedy for enlarged prostate glands accompanied by painful or difficult urination, groin pain, frequent urination, nighttime urination, and fatigue. It is especially effective in the treatment of chronic conditions accompanied by pronounced swelling.

Dose: Kai Kit Wan can be obtained in 54-pill bottles. Take three to six pills two to three times a day.

Hemorrhoids

Fargelin (For Piles)

Fargelin regulates acute or chronic hemorrhoids accompanied by heat signs: these signs include itching, bleeding, burning, prolapse, and constipation. This patent may contain some animal products.

Dose: Fargelin is available in 36- and 60-tablet bottles. Take three tablets three times a day.

See the following pages for treatment of:

Hemorrhoids accompanied by bleeding. Refer to **Yunnan Paiyao** under "Trauma," on page 127.

Gynecological Conditions

Hsiao Yao Wan (Bupleurum Sedative Pills)

This patent is specificically used to treat premenstrual syndrome; menstrual disorders, including cramps, irregular periods, infertility, breast distension, depression, and irritability; vertigo; headaches; fatigue; blurred vision; and red, painful eyes. It also alleviates digestive dysfunction accompanied by abdominal bloating and fullness; hiccups; poor appetite; food allergies; chronic hay fever; and hypoglycemia.

Dose: These pills are available in 100- or 200-pill bottles. Take eight pills three times a day.

Note: This product is also known as *Xiao Yao Wan.*

Butiao Tablets

These tablets effectively treat irregular periods, menstrual pain, excessive uterine bleeding accompanied by fatigue, and anemia.

Dose: Butiao is available in 100-tablet bottles. Take three pills three times a day.

Wu Chi Pai Feng Wan (White Phoenix Pills)

This patent regulates menstrual disorders caused by anemia, including cramps, headaches, amenorrhea, ovulation pain, postpartum weakness, postpartum bleeding, fatigue, lower-back pain, poor appetite, prolonged periods, and irregular periods. *Wu Chi Pai Feng Wan* may also be used to alleviate postpartum fatigue. This medication contains animal products.

Dose: *Wu Chi Pai Feng Wan* is available in 120-pill bottles, or in boxes, each of which contains 10 large chewball pills. Take from one-half to one chewball pill two times a day: chew the pill, or cut it into smaller pieces, and then swallow it. It may also be dissolved in warm water. Take five regular pills three times a day.

Note: A similar formula containing fewer herbs, called *Pai Feng Wan*, is also available.

Tang Kwe Gin

Tang Kwe Gin, a widely used tonic, improves blood quality and builds the blood. It is useful in the treatment of anemia and fatigue resulting from illness, surgery, or trauma. This tonic also regulates palpitations, dizziness, poor memory, irregular menses accompanied by pale blood, amenorrhea, and postpartum weakness resulting from blood loss.

Dose: *Tang Kwe Gin* can be purchased in 100-milliliter, or 200-cc, bottles. Take one to two tablespoons two times a day.

An Tai Wan (For Embryos)

An Tai Wan calms a restless fetus and alleviates premature uterine contractions. It also prevents impending miscarriage (accompanied by lower-abdominal pain) during pregnancy.

Dose: This patent is available in 100-pill bottles. Take seven pills three times a day.

Caution: A qualified practitioner of Traditional Chinese Medicine should monitor use of Chinese herbal patent medicines during pregnancy.

Shih San Tai Pao Wan

Use this patent during the first trimester of pregnancy to prevent miscarriage, fatigue, anemia, and nausea.

Dose: This treatment is available in boxes, each of which contains 10 waxed-egg pills. Take one pill two times a day.

Caution: A qualified practitioner of Traditional Chinese Medicine should monitor use of Chinese herbal patent medicines during pregnancy.

Placenta Compound Restorative Pills (*He Che Da Zao Wan*)

These pills alleviate menopausal night sweats and female hot flashes. It also treats male spermatorrhea in which semen is lost at night, during a dream. Both female and male conditions may be accompanied by dizziness; tinnitus; weak, tired legs; lower-back aches; low-grade afternoon fevers; fatigue; red cheeks; and a hot, flushed face. This patent contains animal products.

Dose: Placenta Compound Restorative is available in 100-pill bottles. Take eight pills three times a day.

See the following pages for treatment of:

Uterine bleeding, repeated miscarriage, uterine prolapse, bladder prolapse, low energy, and digestive weakness. Refer to **Central Qi Pills (Bu Zhong Yi Qi Wan)** under "Energy Tonics," on page 124.

Abnormal uterine bleeding, irregular or heavy menses, palpitations, fatigue, night sweats, insomnia, dizziness, and restless dreaming. Refer to *Gui Pi Wan* under "Restlessness and Insomnia," on page 123.

Impotence, infertility, sexual dysfunction accompanied by coldness in the hands and feet, frequent urination, diarrhea, undigested food in the stools, and fatigue. Refer to **Golden Book Tea (Sexoton Pills)** under "Energy Tonics," on page 125.

Light or irregular menses accompanied by dizziness; poor memory; pale face; and fatigue. Refer to **Eight-Treasure Tea** under "Energy Tonics," on page 124.

Acute vaginitis. Refer to *Yudai Wan* under "Genitourinary Conditions," on page 111.

Severe menstrual cramps and excessive bleeding. Refer to *Yunnan Paiyao* under "Trauma," on page 127.

Menstrual pain. Refer to **Corydalis Yanhusus Analgesic Tablets** under "Pain," on page 127.

Vaginal or menstrual infections, hot flashes, night sweats, burning in the palms of hands or soles of feet, and insomnia. Refer to **Eight-Flavor Tea (Chih Pai Di Huang Wan)** under "Genitourinary Disorders," on page 111.

Digestive Disorders

Ginseng Stomachic Pills (*Ren Shen Jian Pi Wan*)

These pills are used to treat chronic digestion problems accompanied by abdominal bloating and pain; diarrhea; loss of appetite, low energy; a pale face; and an inability to gain or maintain weight.

Dose: Ginseng Stomachic is available in 200-pill bottles. Take six pills three times a day.

Caution: Nursing mothers should not use this patent. Avoid eating cold foods while ingesting Ginseng Stomachic.

Note: This product is commonly available without ginseng, and is also called *Jian Pi Wan*.

Liu Jun Zi Tablets

Liu Jun Zi alleviates poor digestion accompanied by reduced appetite; diarrhea; indigestion; acid regurgitation; and nausea.

Dose: This patent is available in 96-tablet bottles. Take eight tablets three times a day, after meals.

Caution: Avoid eating cold foods while ingesting *Liu Jun Zi*.

Carmichaeli Tea Pills (*Fu Zi Li Zhong Wan*)

These tea pills treats watery, pale diarrhea; nausea; vomiting; poor digestion; pale- to clear-colored urine; abdominal fullness; and cold hands or feet. Carmichaeli Tea Pills contain aconite.

Dose: This patent can be purchased in 200-pill bottles. Take eight to twelve pills three times a day.

Mu Xiang Shun Qi Wan (Aplotaxis Carminative Pills)

This patent regulates food congestion characterized by abdominal distension, poor digestion, erratic stools, constipation, foul-smelling belches, and foul breath. It also treats hypoacidity.

Dose: Mu Xiang Shun Qi Wan is available in 200-pill bottles. Take eight pills two times a day.

Caution: Avoid eating cold foods while ingesting these pills.

Ginseng Royal-Jelly Vials (*Rensheng Feng Wang Jiang*)

This product promotes appetite and stimulates food absorption. It is a beneficial treatment following prolonged illness, surgery, and childbirth; for hypoglycemia; and in old age.

Dose: Ginseng Royal Jelly is available in boxes, each of which contains 10 glass vials; each vial holds 10 cc. Ingest one to two vials per day, either alone or with water. Royal jelly boxes include a glass cutter and straws.

Caution: Do not eat citrus or cold foods, or drink caffeinated beverages while ingesting Gingseng Royal Jelly.

Pill Curing

This treatment alleviates food congestion; food poisoning; stomach flu accompanied by sudden, violent abdominal cramping; bloating characterized by pain; vomiting; headaches; constipation; and diarrhea. It also regulates nausea and motion sickness. Pill Curing is a safe treatment during pregnancy, and for children.

Dose: This patent can be purchased in boxes; each box contains 10 bottles full of pills. Take one to two full bottles as needed.

Ping Wei Pian

Ping Wei Pian treats gastric disturbance, gas, abdominal cramping, abdominal bloating, poor appetite, diarrhea, nausea, and pain. It also maintains the digestive function.

Dose: This patent is available in 48-tablet bottles. Take four tablets two times a day.

Shu Kan Wan (condensed)

This patent regulates abdominal gas, hiccups, belching, flatulence characterized by abdominal pain, poor digestion, loose stools, erratic stools, poor appetite accompanied by nausea, vomiting, regurgitation associated with hyperacidity, cold limbs, and a facial flush.

Dose: Shu Kan Wan can be purchased in 120-pill bottles. Take eight pills three times a day.

Caution: Use of this patent during pregnancy is prohibited.

Fructus Persica Compound Pills

Fructus Persica treats habitual constipation associated with dryness or heat.

Dose: This patent is available in 200-pill bottles. Take four to eight pills three times a day.

Sai Mei An (Internal Formula)

This patent is used to regulate hyperacidity, gastritis associated with stomach hyperacidity, nonbleeding duodenal and gastric ulcers, and stomach irritation and inflammation following meals. *Sai Mei An* also regenerates stomach tissue.

Dose: Sai Mei An is available in 50-pill bottles. Take three pills three times a day, before meals.

Note: Combine this patent with *Yunnan Paiyao* (see "Trauma," on page 127) if bleeding accompanies the symptoms listed above.

Caution: Discontinue use of this patent two weeks after symptoms subside. Long-term use of *Sai Mei An* damages the stomach and digestion.

Wei Te Ling

Wei Te Ling relieves the pain and bleeding associated with gastric and duodenal ulcers, gastritis in conjunction with stomach hyperacidity, stomach distension, and gas.

Dose: This patent can be purchased in 120-tablet bottles. Take four to six tablets three times a day, before meals or when necessary.

See the following pages for treatment of:

Digestive dysfunction accompanied by abdominal bloating, hiccups, poor appetite, and food allergies. Refer to **Hsiao Yao Wan** under "Gynecological Conditions," on page 112.

Poor digestion characterized by abdominal bloating, pain, gas, and erratic stools; chronic diarrhea; hypoglycemia; and low energy. Refer to **Central Qi Pills (Bu Zhong Yi Qi Wan)** under "Energy Tonics," on page 124.

Poor digestion, undigested food in the stools, coldness, lower-back pain, and diarrhea. Refer to **Golden Book Tea (Sexoton Pills)**, under "Energy Tonics," on page 125.

Poor digestion characterized by low appetite, hypoglycemia, a pale face, anemia, fatigue, and dizziness. Refer to **Eight-Treasure Tea** under "Energy Tonics," on page 124.

Stomach pain or gastric or duodenal ulcer pain. Refer to **Corydalis Yanhusus Analgesic Tablets** under "Pain," on page 127.

Poor digestion accompanied by nausea; vertigo; headaches; pasty, loose stools; and flatulence. Refer to **Huo Hsiang Cheng Chi Pien** under "Colds and Flu," on page 103.

Liver and Gallbladder Disorders

Lidan Tablets

This remedy is a specific for acute or chronic gallstone inflammation and bile duct inflammation. It is used to dissolve and remove gallstones.

Dose: Lidan Tablets are available in 120-tablet bottles. Take six tablets three times a day.

Li Gan Pian (Liver Strengthening Tablets)

This patent regulates acute or chronic jaundice, hepatitis, gallstones, and bile. It also decreases liver pain, and can be taken with Lidan Tablets.

Dose: Li Gan Pian is available in 100-tablet bottles. Take two to four tablets three times a day, with meals.

Ji Gu Cao Pills

Ji Gu Cao treats acute or chronic hepatitis accompanied by jaundice, and is reputed to achieve excellent results without side effects. To treat acute hepatitis, combine this patent with Li Gan Pian (see above).

Dose: This patent can be purchased in 50-pill bottles. Take four pills three times a day.

See the following pages for treatment of:

Hepatitis or gallbladder pain. See **Corydalis Yanhusus Analgesic Tablets** under "Pain," on page 127.

Heart Disorders

Danshen Tabletco

This patent treats angina pectoris accompanied by left-arm pain; heart palpitations; and chest pains. It also reduces blood cholesterol and lipids.

Dose: *Danshen* Tabletco is available in 50-pill bottles. Take three pills three times a day.

Caution: If an individual suffers from the symptoms listed above, s/he should seek the aid of a qualified health practitioner.

Ren Shen Zai Zao Wan (Ginseng Restorative Pills)

Ren Shen Zai Zao Wan alleviates stroke-related symptoms, including hemiplegia; speech disturbances; and contractive, spastic, or flaccid muscle tone in the extremities. It is also effectively treats facial paralysis (Bell's palsy). This remedy contains some animal products.

Dose: This patent is available in boxes, each of which contains 10 pills held in wax eggs. It can also be purchased in 50-pill bottles. Take 1 wax-egg pill twice a day or 10 bottle pills once a day.

Caution: Use of Ren Shen Zai Zao Wan during pregnancy is prohibited. Do not use this treatment in the presence of bleeding.

See the following pages for treatment of:

Stroke-related paralysis, Bell's palsy accompanied by migraines, and rheumatic pain. Refer to **Tian Ma Wan** under "Arthritis and Rheumatism," on page 121.

Skin Disorders

Margarite Acne Pills

These pills treat acne (particularly adolescent acne), furuncles, skin itching, rashes, and hives.

Dose: This patent is available in 30-pill bottles. Take six pills two times a day.

Caution: Reduce this medication's dosage if diarrhea develops.

Lien Chiao Pai Tu Pien

Lien Chiao Pai Tu Pien alleviates acute inflammations and infections of ulcerated abscesses and carbuncles accompanied by pus, and skin itching characterized by rashes and redness.

Dose: This patent is available in boxes, each of which contains 12 vials; each vial holds eight tablets. Take two to four tablets twice a day.

Caution: Use of this treatment during pregnancy is prohibited.

See the following pages for treatment of:

Furuncles and abscesses: Refer to **Chuan Xin Lian** under "Sore Throats, Mouth Disorders, and Ear Problems," on page 108.

Ulcerative skin lesions. Refer to **Superior Sore Throat Powder Spray** under "Sore Throats, Mouth Disorders, and Ear Problems," on page 109.

Itching and hives. Refer to **Huang Lien Shang Ching Pien** under "Sore Throats, Mouth Disorders, and Ear Problems," on page 108.

Boils, nose sores, mouth sores, toothaches, sore throat, and nosebleeds. Refer to **Ching Fei Yi Huo Pian** under "Coughing, Phlegm, and Labored Breathing," on page 104.

Arthritis and Rheumatism

Specific Lumbaglin

This patent relieves inflammation, lower-back pain, muscular strain, and sciatic inflammation. It also alleviates waist and kidney pain.

Dose: This treatment is available in 24-capsule boxes. Take one to two capsules three times a day.

Caution: Avoid use of this patent during pregnancy. Also, do not consume beans and seafood while taking this medication.

Du Huo Jisheng Wan

This classic Chinese formula regulates lower-back and knee pain accompanied by cold-induced weakness, stiffness, and numbness; frequent, clear-colored urination; nighttime urination; sensations of cold; and aversions to cold. Conditions with this symptomology include chronic sciatica, arthritis, and rheumatism.

Dose: Du Huo Jisheng Wan can be purchased in 100-pill bottles. Take nine pills twice a day.

Caution: Avoid use of this treament during pregnancy. Also, do not consume beans, seafood, or cold food while taking this medication.

Xiao Huo Luo Dan

This patent treats rheumatic pain; numbness; difficult joint movement; sharp joint pain; joint or muscle aches; chronic, cold-induced lower-back pain; frequent, clear-colored urination; nighttime urination; sensations of cold; and aversions to cold.

Dose: Xiao Huo Luo Dan is available in 100-pill bottles. Take six pills two to three times a day.

Caution: Use of this patent during pregnancy is prohibited. Do not use Xiao Huo Luo Dan in the presence of red, swollen joints or fever. Also, do not consume beans, seafood, or cold food while taking this medication.

Feng Shih Hsiao Tung Wan

Use this patent to alleviate rheumatism characterized by lower-back aches; chronic sciatica; and fingers, shoulder, knee, or hip pain accompanied by a sensation of cold in the limbs. It is a preferred treatment for chronic rheumatoid arthritis, osteoarthritis, and geriatric leg debility.

Dose: This treatment is available in 100-pill bottles. Take 10 pills twice a day.

Caution: Avoid use of Feng Shih Hsiao Tung Wan during pregnancy. Also, do not consume beans, seafood, or cold food while taking this medication.

Tian Ma Wan

Tian Ma Wan alleviates rheumatic or arthritic pain accompanied by sensations of cold; migraines; face, arm, or leg paralysis; and Bell's palsy. It is an excellent treatment for the elderly.

Dose: This patent can be purchased in 100-pill bottles. Take six to eight pills three times a day.

See the following pages for treatment of:

Rheumatic pain. Refer to **Corydalis Yanhusus Analgesic Tablets** under "Pain," on page 127.

Rheumatism characterized by difficult movement, painful joints, numbness, and tingling limbs. Refer to **Ren Shen Zai Zao Wan** under "Heart Disorders," on page 119.

Restlessness and Insomnia

An Mien Pien

An Mien Pien regulates insomnia accompanied by mental agitation or exhaustion; anxiety; red or irritated eyes; excessive dreaming; overthinking;

and poor memory.

Dose: This patent is available in 60-tablet bottles. Take four tablets three times a day.

Caution: Do not consume hot, greasy foods while taking this medication.

Ding Xin Wan

This patent treats restlessness, anxiety, insomnia, palpitations, poor memory, dizziness, hot flashes, and dry mouth.

Dose: Ding Xin Wan can be purchased in 100-pill bottles. Take six pills two to three times a day.

Caution: Do not consume hot, greasy foods while taking this medication.

Emperor's Tea (*Tian Wang Bu Xin Wan*)

This tea alleviates insomnia, restlessness, anxiety, palpitations, vivid dreaming, and nocturnal emissions accompanied by night sweats. It may be used to treat hyperactive thyroid conditions. Emperor's Tea is also an excellent aid for students during prolonged studying, which depletes the heart blood and *yin,* causing the above-named symptoms.

Dose: This product is available in 200-pill bottles. Take eight pills three times a day.

Caution: Do not drink this tea for longer than two weeks at a time. Discontinue its use for one week and then resume ingestion for another two weeks. Also, do not consume hot, greasy foods while taking this medication.

Shen Ching Shuai Jao Wan

This patent treats insomnia, nightmares, restless sleep, night sweats, vertigo, tinnitus, palpitations, and fatigue. It contains some animal products.

Dose: Shen Ching Shuai Jao Wan can be purchased in 200-pill bottles. Take 20 pills twice a day.

Caution: Excessive or prolonged use of *Shen Ching Shuai Jao Wan* can impair the digestion. Discontinue its use after two weeks and then resume ingestion after another two weeks have passed. Also, do not consume cold foods while taking this medication.

An Sheng Bu Xin Wan

An Sheng Bu Xin Wan alleviates insomnia, palpitations, poor memory, uneasiness, excessive dreaming, restlessness, and dizziness. It is a calming, soothing, and tranquilizing treatment.

Dose: This patent is available in 300-pill bottles. Take 15 pills three times a day.

Caution: Discontinue its use after two weeks and then resume ingestion after another two weeks have passed.

Gui Pi Wan (Kwei Be Wan)

This patent regulates insomnia, palpitations, dizziness, nightmares, restless dreaming, poor memory, fatigue, and night sweats. It also effectively treats irregular menstrual cycles and abnormal uterine bleeding.

Dose: Gui Pi Wan is available in 200-pill bottles. Take eight pills three times a day.

See the following pages for treatment of:

Insomnia caused by pain. Refer to **Corydalis *Yanhusus* Analgesic Tablets** under "Pain," on page 127.

Hypertension

Compound Cortex Eucommia Tablets (*Fu Fang Du Zhong Pian*)

These tablets regulate hypertension characterized by a flushed or pale face, sensations of cold, lower-back pain, palpitations, headaches, dizziness, frequent urination, and fatigue.

Dose: This patent is available in 100-tablet bottles. Take five tablets three times a day.

Caution: Do not eat cold foods while taking these tablets.

Hypertension Repressing Tablets (*Jiang Ya Ping Pian*)

This patent treats hypertension characterized by dizziness, tinnitus, and headaches; and a flushed face accompanied by heat signs, including thirst, yellow phlegm, dark-yellow urine, and constipation. It may also be used to lower blood cholesterol and prevent hardening of the arteries. After using this patent, hypertension should be reduced within two weeks. This formula can be used for several years without causing side effects. It contains some animal products.

Dose: These tablets are available in boxes, each of which contains 12 bottles. Each bottle holds 12 tablets. Take four tablets three times a day, in three 14-day consecutive courses.

Caution: Do not eat hot, greasy foods while taking this medication.

See the following pages for treatment of:

Hypertension accompanied by tinnitus, thirst, eye irritation, and pressure; insomnia, and headaches. Refer to **Tso-Tzu Otic Pills** under "Sore Throats, Mouth Disorders, and Ear Problems," on page 109.

Energy Tonics

Central Qi Pills (*Bu Zhong Yi Qi Wan*)

This pill combination regulates low energy; poor digestion with abdominal bloating, pain, gas, and erratic stools; and rectal, uterinary, colonic, hemorrhoidal, varicose-vein, and hernial prolapse. It also prevents uterine bleeding, repeated miscarriages, chronic diarrhea, and hypoglycemia.

Dose: Central *Qi* Pills are available in 100-pill bottles. Take eight pills three times a day.

Caution: This patent should not be used in the presence of heat; aversion to heat; thirst; profuse sweating; strong body odor; dark-yellow, scant urine; or yellow-to-red discharges. Also, do not eat cold foods while ingesting these pills.

Eight-Treasure Tea

This classical formula nourishes the blood and strengthens energy. It is an excellent general tonic, particularly for women who exhibit the following symptoms: pale face, fatigue, dizziness, shortness of breath, heart palpitations, anemia, hypoglycemia, low appetite, irregular menstruation, amenorrhea, or general weakness during pregnancy. It also facilitates recovery from childbirth or illness.

Dose: This product can be purchased in 200-pill bottles. Take eight pills three times a day.

Golden Book Tea (Sexoton Pills)

This pill formula treats lowered energy characterized by coldness; lower-back aches; poor digestion characterized by gas or undigested food in stools; persistent diarrhea; poor circulation; frequent, clear urination; edema; impotence; infertility; and lowered sex drive.

Dose: This product is available in 120-pill and 200-pill bottles. Take eight to ten pills three times a day.

Caution: Not to be taken by those with heat, an aversion to heat, thirst, or yellow discharges, or phlegm. Avoid eating cold foods.

Six-Flavor Tea (*Liu Wei Di Huang Wan*)

Six-Flavor Tea regulates lowered energy, as characterized by sore throats, thirst, mild night sweats, dizziness, burning sensations in soles of feet or palms of hands, impotence, tinnitis, restlessness, insomnia, and lower-back pain.

Dose: This patent is available in 200-pill bottles. Take eight to twelve pills three times a day.

Yang Rong Wan (Ginseng Tonic Pills)

Yang Rong Wan promotes and maintains health and longevity. These pills effectively treat general weakness caused by chronic illnesses, childbirth, surgery, or trauma.

Dose: This patent can be obtained in 200-pill bottles. Take eight pills three times a day.

Caution: *Yang Rong Wan* should not be taken in the presence of heat, aversion to heat, thirst, or yellow discharges, or phlegm. Also, do not eat cold foods while taking this medication.

See the following pages for treatment of:

Fatigue accompanied by dizziness, palpitations, irregular menses, amenorrhea, poor memory, and anemia. Refer to **Tang Kwe Gin** under "Gynecological Conditions," on page 113.

Fatigue accompanied by dizziness, palpitations, irregular menses, poor memory, night sweats, insomnia, and abnormal uterine bleeding. Refer to **Gui Pi Wan** under "Restlessness and Insomnia," on page 123.

Pediatric Disorders

Bo Ying Pills

These pills regulate a wide range of pediatric diseases, including fever, difficult respiration, productive coughing, teething, stomachache, diarrhea, vomiting, restlessness, and night crying. It contains some animal products.

Dose: Bo Ying is available in tins; each tin holds six vials of powder. This patent may be mixed with food or placed on the mother's nipple, in the following dosages: 0 to 1 month, 1/2 bottle one to two times a day; 1 month to 3 years, 1 bottle, one to two times a day; 3 to 10 years, 2 to 3 bottles, one to two times a day. A preventative dose may be taken twice a month.

Caution: Use of Bo Ying should be restricted to one to two doses a day for no more than three to five days at a time.

Hui Chun Tan

Hui Chun Tan treats fever, coughing accompanied by phlegm, colds, restlessness, measles, stomachaches, vomiting, diarrhea, and difficult respiration. It contains some animal products.

Dose: This patent can be purchased in boxes, each of which contain 10 bottles. Each bottle holds three pills. It should be taken in the following dosages: 0 to 1 year, take 1 pill three times a day; 1 to 5 years, take 3 pills three times a day; 5 to 9 years, take 5 pills three times a day

Caution: Use of Hui Chun Tan should be restricted to one to two doses a day for no more than three to five days at a time.

Tao Chih Pien (For Babies)

This patent treats children aged one month to seven years. It relieves sore throats; mouth sores; swollen gums; fever; reddened eyes; constipation; stomachaches; and scant, dark urine. It contains some animal products.

Dose: Tao Chih Pien can be purchased in boxes; there are 12 tubes (each of which contains eight tablets) in each box. It should be taken in the following dosages: 0 to 1 year, one to two tablets twice a day; one to seven years, two to four tablets twice a day.

Caution: Use of Tao Chih Pien should be restricted to one to two doses over a short period of time. Reduce or discontinue use of this patent if diarrhea develops.

See the following pages for treatment of:

Acute tonsillitis, acute mumps, and strep throat. Refer to **Laryngitis Pills** under "Sore Throats, Mouth Disorders, and Ear Problems," on page 108.

Pain

Corydalis *Yanhusus* Analgesic Tablets

These tablets regulate dysmenorrhea pain, postpartum pain, stomachaches, gastric- or duodenal-ulcer pain, abdominal pain, pained caused by hepatitis, gallbladder pain, chest pain, pain caused by rheumatism or injury, and insomnia caused by pain. Additionally, it effectively treats tremors, spasms, and seizures.

Dose: Corydalis *Yanhusus* is available in 20-tablet bottles. Take four to six pills three times a day or as needed.

Trauma

Yunnan Paiyao

This patent, formulated primarily from the *tien qi* ginseng root, stops internal and external bleeding; pain caused by wounds, cuts, and hemorrhages; bloody vomit; bloody stools; expectoration of blood; serious nosebleeds; and excessive menstrual bleeding. It eases traumatic swelling caused by injuries, including fractures, sprains, ligament tears, muscle tears, dislocations, bone breaks, and bruising resulting from falls or blows. *Yunnan Paiyao* also treats excessive menstrual bleeding, severe menstrual cramps, ulcer bleeding, insect bites, and carbuncles. It may be taken internally or applied externally.

Dose: Yunnan Paiyao can be purchased in boxes, each of which contains 10 bottles. Each bottle holds 4 grams of powder. It is also available in 20-capsule packets. For internal use, take .2 to .5 grams (or one to two capsules) four times a day. For external use, apply this patent directly to bleeding wounds. With deep or wide wounds, hold the sides of the cut together, pour the powder over the wound, and keep it closed for one to two minutes. In all external applications, clean the wound first and bandage it after the patent has been applied.

Caution: Internal use of *Yunnan Paiyao* during pregnancy is prohibited.

Zheng Gu Shui

This external-use-only liniment relieves pain; relaxes tendons and muscles; and promotes healing from traumatic injuries, including fractures, sprains, dislocated joints, ligament and muscle tears, and bruising. It is an effective treatment for sports and martial-arts injuries.

Dose: Zheng Gu Shui is available in 30 cc and 100 cc bottles. Apply this linament during light massage or with gauze. It will stain clothes, but it can be removed with rubbing alcohol.

Caution: This patent should not enter the eyes. Those who apply Zheng Gu Shui should wash their hands thoroughly after use. Keep this volatile linament away from flame. Do not rub Zheng Gu Shui into open wounds. Discontinue use of this linament if a serious skin reaction occurs.

See the following pages for treatment of:

Pain caused by trauma or injury. Refer to **Corydalis Yanhusus Analgesic Tablets** under "Pain," on page 127.

Chinese Herbal Diet

An appropriate diet is essential to regaining and maintaining the body's health. Just as each herb has a particular heating or cooling energy, food warms or cools the body. Warming foods aid metabolism and circulate blood, while cooling foods slow the metabolism and cool the body. Over time, excessive consumption of heating foods causes the body to become hot, while excessive consumption of cooling foods causes the body to become cold.

It is vital to choose foods according to their heating or cooling energies. If you take herbs appropriate to your condition but eat foods with the wrong energy, then you will receive little or no benefit from the herbs. Thus, it is very important to eat an appropriate energetic diet while taking herbs. Furthermore, consuming food appropriate to your body's energy helps prevent illnesses from setting in.

Digestion

Digestion can be compared to a pot of bubbling soup on the stove. When we add foods directly from the refrigerator or freezer to the soup, the soup stops bubbling and it takes a while to regain a boil. We can assist the boiling process by turning up the burner under the pot. If cooling foods are added over a period of time, however, we can't turn the heat up any longer. The fires have cooled, dampened, and become dim, and we have to wait until the soup begins to boil again.

Similarly, if we consume too many cooling foods or drinks directly from the refrigerator or freezer, our bodies will try to turn up our inner burners. This process can generate excessive heat, which manifests itself as headaches across the forehead, bleeding gums, bad breath, and stomach hyperacidity.

In time, the body becomes incapable of turning up the inner burners any higher. Instead, it metabolizes food poorly, especially cooling foods. Eventually, the digestion becomes so cold that food cannot be sufficiently broken down. Undigested food, which can be seen in the stool, begins to pass through the body. When digestion becomes cold, it is incapable of breaking down food and fluids, and of assimilating nutrients. Over time, fatigue, lowered immunity, and anemia result.

Conversely, if you add hot foods to a recently heated soup, it boils harder and faster, causing spurts of fluid or oil to jump out of the pot. Excessive consumption of hot, greasy foods—either taken directly from the stove or oven, or those with a heating energy—creates the same effect, and may lead to headaches, hypertension, irritability, restlessness, insomnia, hyperacidity, hyperactivity, thirst, infections, inflammations, and numerous other diseases. Once again, it is critical to select foods according to their energies.

The Energy of Food

A balanced diet is primarily comprised of foods with neutral-to-slightly-warm and slightly-cool energies. Grains and legumes are neutral; fish, chicken, beef, and pork are slightly warm; and cooked vegetables and some fruits are slightly cool.

Hot, greasy foods or foods with excessive heat include: caffeine in all of its forms, as found in coffee, black tea, cocoa, colas, and chocolate; alcohol; nuts; nut butters; cheese; fried, fatty foods; chips; avocados; turkey; and lamb. Raw foods, salads, most fruits, iced drinks, foods and drinks eaten directly from the refrigerator or freezer, and diets containing deficient protein and fats are excessively cooling.

Ideally, the food you consume should be organic and unprocessed. Processed foods convert quickly into sugar, have few nutrients, and lead to congestion. Ingestion of toxic foods such as white sugar, white salt, caffeine, and alcohol should be kept at a minimum. These substances quickly imbalance the body and cause disease. Often, symptoms are cured simply by eliminating these foods from the diet.

Therapeutic Use of Food

When treating a heat-related illness, it is important to eat cooling foods and eliminate hot, greasy foods. Cooling foods are eaten until the illness is healed and the body is brought back into balance. A balanced diet should be adopted after symptoms subside. The continued consumption of cooling foods—such as salads, raw foods, and fruit juices—will eventually cause another imbalance in the body, and create coldness.

It is common for individuals suffering from heat, as caused by excessive meat eating, to adopt a vegetarian or raw-food diet and feel great for a while. Continued consumption of these foods, however, creates coldness. The symptomology of coldness includes: emaciation, lowered immunity, fatigue, clear-to-white bodily secretions, undigested food in the stools, diarrhea, frequent and copious urination, poor appetite, and sensations of coldness. Thus, it is very important to adopt a balanced diet once the illness has been healed.

When treating a cold-related illness, it is vital to eat warming foods and avoid cooling ones. Individuals with cold-related illnesses should eat cooked foods and avoid raw substances, salads, fruit and vegetable juices, and anything taken directly from the refrigerator or freezer. Protein-rich and warm-natured foods should also be consumed with every meal.

Vegetarians with excessive bodily coolness must eat a much stricter diet to regain and maintain balance in the body. In this case, diets should be limited to cooked foods with sufficient protein and seasoned with spices such as cumin, coriander, garlic, and onions. These spices are warming and help the digestion. Adopt a balanced diet once symptoms are healed.

The Chinese have identified the specific therapeutic energies of most foods. They use foods with particular energies in specific recipes; these foods help alleviate illness and strengthen various organ complexes. Several books delineate food's therapeutic properties and list recipes used to treat various ailments. For a list of these books, refer to "Recommended Reading and Sources," on page 188.

Protein

Recent research shows that individual protein needs are based on ancestry, blood type, and metabolism. Protein needs also vary according to types of work performed; mental work creates a higher protein demand, while physical work generates a need for complex carbohydrates.

As a general rule, protein should be consumed with every meal. Beans with grains or small amounts of animal products generally contain appropriate amounts of protein. Protein needs are highly individual. Do not adopt generalized, popular diets; instead, discover a balanced diet that suits your body's needs.

Cooking with Herbs

One of the best ways to strengthen the body is to consume herbs cooked with food. Herbs cooked with food are highly digestible, assimilable, extremely nutritious, and sometimes delicious. Herbs often appear in soups and congees.

Cooking with Chinese herbs can be simple: lycii berries can be substituted for raisins in hot cereal or oatmeal cookies, and a few sticks of astragalus can be added to cooking grains. This healthful cuisine can also be more creative, as when highly nutritious soup stocks are made with specific herbal formulas. Astragalus, jujube dates, Chinese wild yam, lycii berries, lotus seeds, and lily stamen are commonly used in soup stocks.

Herbs should be soaked for several hours and then added (with the water in which they were soaked) to cooking soup. If time does not permit, however, they can be soaked for a shorter period of time or not at all. Many cooked herbs can be eaten with the soup, and are quite delicious. If an herb hasn't been soaked, ensure that it is well cooked before consuming it—it should be easy to chew and swallow. Fibrous or unpleasant-tasting herbs can be strained out and discarded. The following recipes indicate whether to eat or discard the herbs.

Soups

Many Chinese typically prepare an herbal soup once a week. Particular herbs are used according to the season, the current weather, and family members' health needs. Some soups are continuously cooked with various scraps added over time. These scraps may include bones, eggshells, and vegetable cuttings. Small amounts of vinegar, which help pull calcium out of bones and shells, are also added. The resulting soup is eventually strained and cooked down to a thick, black, gel-like substance, which is used in small amounts to season soups or stir-frys. It is highly nutritious and laden with minerals and vitamins. This type of cooking is also a part of traditional European and Native American cultures.

Preparing Soups

We can easily prepare a soup stock similar to the one described above by cooking vegetable peelings and eggshells, which are stored in the freezer until you are ready to use them, over low heat in a pot of water with or without bones. Oxtail or other bones, ribs, or meat can be added to the mixture. Herbs are also added, and everything is cooked together. The resulting mixture is strained and meat can be reintroduced, if desired.

A simple stock is made into soup by cooking herbs in water and then adding grains, vegetables, beans, or meat. Cooked herbs in water can be saved and used alone as stock for grains, cereals, or soups. When adding meat, cool the finished soup overnight, so fat can be skimmed off in the morning. If desired, add one to two tablespoons of miso (soybean paste), which helps blend the flavors and mask any unusual herbal taste.

Basic Soup Recipe
(serves four people)

3 1/2 quarts of water
1 cup of rice or other grains
1 cup of lentils, or 8 ounces of meat
2 cups of vegetables
2 ounces of Chinese herbs, as desired
1 tablespoon of vinegar, if bones are included

When using bones: Make a stock from bones, vegetable peelings, or eggshells by simmering these substances with vinegar, for three hours. Add herbs and cook the resulting mix for another 30 minutes. Strain the stock and reintroduce meat and the edible herbs. Add rice and vegetables, and simmer for 30 to 45 minutes.

When using herbs exclusively: Simmer Chinese herbs, vegetable peelings, or eggshells (add vinegar if eggshells are included) for 30 minutes. Strain the resulting mixture and add any additional ingredients, including edible herbs. Simmer for 45 minutes.

Sample Soup Recipes

To make a complete meal, add rice and vegetables to the following basic soup recipes.

Bone Marrow Soup

This traditional soup builds blood and strengthens Essence, bones, and kidneys. It effectively treats anemia, insufficient menses, paleness, dizziness, weakness, fatigue, lower-back pain, and weakened eyesight and hearing.

Pork ribs or oxtail bones

Chinese herbs as desired, including *dang gui*, lycii berries, astragalus, Chinese
    yam, or cooked rehmannia

Seasonings, as desired

Cook bones or ribs in large pot of water for 3.5 hours, and skim off the dirty foam that arises during the first hour of preparation. Add herbs and cook for another 30 minutes. Strain, and reintroduce meat, if desired, and edible herbs. Add desired seasonings. Let the resulting mixture cool, and scrape fat off the top. Eat this soup as is, or use it as a broth base with which to cook grains or cereals. Small portions of this soup can be frozen. Consume one bowl daily, to strengthen the blood and body.

Chinese Yam and Lycii Berry Soup

(serves four people)

This soup strengthens digestion, lungs, liver, and kidneys. It also treats diabetes and strengthens eyesight.

1/2 pound of any lean meat (beef is ideal)
1 ounce of Chinese yam
1 ounce of lycii berries

Cook Chinese yam and lycii berries in water, with meat, and add grains and vegetables if desired. These herbs may be eaten with the soup.

Dang Gui and Lamb Soup

(serves four people)

This soup warms the body, builds blood and energy, strengthens digestion, and treats menstrual pain and insufficiency. Traditionally, it is eaten by women for three days after each menstrual cycle and after childbirth. Women who have stopped bleeding may eat this soup ritually, once a month, to strengthen their blood.

1 ounce of *dang gui*
1/2 pound of lamb
Ginger slices to taste

Cook lamb and *dang gui* together, until lamb is tender. Add the ginger slices during the last 15 minutes of preparation. *Dang gui* is bitter; it can be removed before the soup is consumed.

Loranthus and Egg Soup
(serves one person)

This soup relieves liver and kidney complaints, impending miscarriage, rheumatism, back pain, loss of sensation in the limbs, diabetes, high blood pressure caused by arteriosclerosis, and back pain in pregnant women. It also promotes breast milk; prevents illness; nourishes skin, muscles, and hair; and strengthens teeth.

2 eggs
1 ounce of loranthus

Make loranthus tea in 12 ounces of water and strain it. Crack eggs into the tea and then hard-boil them. Eat the eggs and drink the tea.

Lotus Seed, Lily, and Pork Soup
(serves four people)

This soup strengthens the digestion and kidneys; promotes mental stability; and heals dry coughing, tuberculosis, neurasthenia, leukorrhea, diarrhea, seminal emissions, wet dreams, and excessive menstrual loss.

8 ounces of lean pork
3/4 ounce of lotus seeds
1 ounce of lily bulb

Cook lean pork in water for two hours. Add herbs, grains, and vegetables (if desired) and cook the resulting mixture for 45 minutes. Herbs may be eaten with the rest of the soup.

Kidneys with Eucommia Soup
(serves two people)

This soup treats back pain, lowers blood pressure and cholesterol, and prevents impending miscarriage during the middle stages of pregnancy. It strengthens the kidneys, liver, tendons, and bones.

4 kidneys (preferably pig kidneys)
1 ounce of eucommia

Make eucommia tea in two cups of water. Strain the tea and add it, along with kidneys and any other desired ingredients, to the soup. Cook the resulting mixture until kidneys are done.

Chicken with He Shou Wu Soup
(serves four people)

Chicken and he shou wu soup nourishes the blood and strengthens the kidneys. It also effectively relieves uterine and hemorrhoidal problems, and keeps hair shiny and its normal color.

1 ounce he shou wu (Polygonum multiflorum)
1 small chicken

Extract internal organs from the chicken. Grind the he shou wu to a powder in a coffee grinder, nut-and-seed grinder, or blender. Wrap the resulting powder in several layers of muslin. Place the muslin inside the chicken, and boil the chicken in water until its meat falls away from the bones. Remove the packet of powdered herbs and bones. Add salt, oil, ginger, and wine (to taste) to the soup. Drink the soup and eat the chicken.

Heart Soup
(serves four people)

This soup nourishes the heart, promotes blood circulation, calms the Spirit, aids mental clarity and sleep, and reduces hypertension.

Use lamb to treat the following symptoms: palpitations, cold hands and feet, aversion to cold, dizziness, poor memory, anxiety, a tendency to be startled, pale lips, and insomnia.

Use mung beans to treat the following symptoms: palpitations, mental restlessness, uneasiness, malar flush, sensations of heat (especially in the evening, night sweats, dry mouth and throat, thirst, mouth and tongue ulcers, dark-yellow urine, agitation, a bitter taste in the mouth, and insomnia.

8 cups of water
1/2 ounce of reishi mushroom
3/4 ounce of longan berries
6 pitted jujube dates
1/2 ounce of lily bulb
1/2 ounce of lotus seeds
1/4 ounce of carthamus
8 ounces of lamb (organic, if possible), or one-half cup of mung beans (washed and with stones removed)
1/2 cup of raw corn
1/4 cup of wheat berries
1 small eggplant
1/2 cup of beets
1/2 cup of carrots
1/2 cup of greens (collard, kale, or mustard)
Salt and sesame seeds (to taste)
1 tablespoon of toasted sesame oil

When using meat: Cook wheat berries with six cups water for one hour. Cook reishi mushroom (in a separate pot) in two cups of water for 45 minutes. Add carthamus and simmer the mixture for 15 minutes. Strain the reishi and carthamus tea and discard the herbs. Add tea, lamb, corn (if it's fresh), and the remaining herbs to the wheat-berries-and-water mixture, and cook it for 30 minutes. Add chopped vegetables and corn (if it's frozen or canned) and cook the resulting mixture for another 15 minutes. Herbs may be eaten with the soup.

When using beans: Soak the beans in six cups of water for eight hours, then cook them with wheat berries for one hour and 15 minutes. Cook reishi mushroom in two cups of water for 45 minutes. Add carthamus and simmer the mixture for 15 minutes. Strain the reishi and carthamus tea and discard the herbs. Add tea, corn (if it's fresh), and the remaining herbs to mung beans and wheat berries, and cook the resulting mixture for 30 minutes. Add the chopped vegetables and corn (if it's frozen or canned), and cook everything for another 15 minutes. Herbs may be eaten with the soup.

Spleen Soup
(serves four people)

Spleen soup strengthens the digestion, appetite, and energy; alleviates gas and bloatedness; and counteracts diarrhea.

Use beef to treat the following symptoms: poor appetite, abdominal bloating after eating, fatigue, weakness of the arms and legs, loose stools, undigested food in the stools, edema, chilliness, cold hands and feet, tiredness, and lack of thirst.

Use beans to treat the following symptoms: lack of appetite, thirst accompanied by a desire to drink in small sips, nausea, loose stools with an offensive odor, scant and dark-yellow urination, and headaches. Omit codonopsis from recipe and substitute 1/2 ounce of chrysanthemum when beans are used.

8 cups of water
2 codonopsis roots or 1/2 ounce of chrysanthemum
1/2 ounce of Chinese yam
7 pitted red dates
1/2 ounce of *fu ling*
8 ounces of lean beef (organic, if possible), or 1/2 cup of garbanzo or aduki beans
1 small yam or sweet potato
1 cup of carrots
1 cup of string beans
Dried ginger and cardamom (to taste)

When using meat: Cook the meat with grain, in water, for 15 minutes. Add the herbs, except for chrysanthemum, and cook the resulting mixture for 15 minutes. Add the chopped vegetables and cook for an additional 15 minutes. Finally, add seasonings. Herbs may be eaten with the rest of the soup.

When using beans: Soak the beans in seven cups of water for eight hours, then cook them in water for one hour and 15 minutes. Simmer the chrysanthemum in one cup of water for 15 minutes. Strain out the herb and add the remaining tea to the beans. Add the grain and cook the resulting mixture for 15 minutes. Add the herbs (with the exception of codonopsis) and cook for another 15 minutes. Add the chopped vegetables and cook everything for an additional 15 minutes. Finally, add seasonings. Herbs may be eaten with the rest of the soup.

Lung Soup
(*serves four people*)

This soup nourishes lungs, eliminates phlegm, and assists breathing.

Use duck to treat the following symptoms: night sweats, insomnia, dry mouth and throat, dry coughing characterized by sticky phlegm, malar flush, heat in the palms of hands and the soles of feet, and shortness of breath.

Use chicken to treat the following symptoms: shortness of breath, coughing accompanied by watery or white phlegm, a weak voice, daytime sweating, aversion to speech, aversion to cold, frequent colds and flu, and tiredness.

Use black beans to treat the following symptoms: coughing accompanied by yellow or green phlegm, shortness of breath, thirst, and swollen tonsils.

8 cups of water
3 sticks of astragalus
1/2 ounce of American-ginseng root
1/2 ounce of glehnia
1/2 ounce of almond or apricot seeds
1/4 ounce of tangerine peel
8 ounces of duck or chicken (organic, if possible), or 1/2 cup of black beans
1 fresh pear
1/2 cup of rice
1/2 cup of sautéed onions (red or yellow)
3 cloves of garlic
1 cup of water chestnuts
1 cup of carrots
1 cup of mustard greens
1/2 cup of walnuts
1 tablespoon of grated fresh ginger
Salt, black pepper, and chopped parsley (to taste)

When using meat: Cook the meat, in water, for 15 minutes. Add rice to the meat and water, and cook 15 minutes. Add herbs (place the tangerine peel in a muslin bag) to this mixture and cook it for 15 minutes. Add sautéed onions and garlic, vegetables, walnuts, and the pear, and cook the resulting mixture for 15 minutes. Add seasonings. Remove the tangerine peel and astragalus.

When using beans: Soak the beans in water eight hours, then cook them for one hour and 15 minutes. Add the rice to the beans and water, and cook the resulting mixture for 15 minutes. Add herbs (place the tangerine peel in a muslin bag) and cook for 15 minutes. Add sautéed onions and garlic, vegetables, walnuts, and the pear and cook the resulting mixture for 15 minutes. Add seasonings. Remove the tangerine peel and astragalus.

Kidney Soup
(serves four people)

This soup strengthens the kidneys. It also helps alleviate frequent or nighttime urination, lower-back pain, poor memory, fatigue, lowered sex drive, and weak knees.

Use pork to treat the following symptoms: lower-back pain, a sensation of cold in the back, cold and weak knees, aversion to cold, impotence, lassitude, abundant and clear urination, scant urination, infertility, loose stools, dizziness, night sweats, nighttime dry mouth, thirst, nocturnal emissions, and chronic vaginal discharge.

Use beans to treat the following symptoms: loose stools, leg and ankle edema, lower-back and knee soreness and weakness, dribbling after urination, urinary incontinence, and chronic vaginal discharge.

8 cups of water
1/4 ounce of he shou wu (*Polygonum multiflorum*)
1/2 ounce of Chinese yam
1/2 ounce of rehmannia
1/4 ounce of cornus
1/4 ounce of alisma
8 ounces of pork (organic, if possible), or 1/2 cup of aduki or kidney beans
1/2 cup of rice or millet
1 six-inch strip of kombu seaweed
1 cup of asparagus (fresh, if possible)
1 cup of string beans
1 cup of celery
1/2 cup of walnuts
1 tablespoon of toasted sesame oil
Parsley, cinnamon, and black sesame seeds (to taste)

When using pork: Cook the pork in four cups of water for one hour. Simmer the *he shou wu*, rehmannia, alisma, and cornus in four cups of water for 30 minutes. Remove and discard the herbs. Add the grain, Chinese yam, and herb tea to the pork, and cook the resulting mixture for 30 minutes. Add the chopped vegetables and walnuts, and cook everything for 15 minutes. Finally, add seasonings.

When using beans: Soak the beans for eight hours in four cups of water, then cook them for one hour and 15 minutes. Simmer the *he shou wu*, rehmannia, alisma, and cornus in four cups of water for 30 minutes. Remove and discard the herbs. Add the grain, Chinese yam, and herb tea to the beans, and cook the resulting mixture for 30 minutes. Add the chopped vegetables and walnuts and cook everything for 15 minutes. Finally, add seasonings.

Liver Soup
(*serves four people*)

This soup harmonizes the liver function, builds blood, clears heat in the liver, and aids eyesight. It also alleviates reddened eyes, menstrual difficulty, premenstrual syndrome, mood swings, hypertension, and the effects of stress.

Use meat to treat the following symptoms: limb numbness, blurred vision, "floaters" in the eyes, amenorrhea (scant menstruation, pale lips, muscle weakness or spasms, cramps, withered and brittle nails, insomnia, night sweats, and nighttime dry throat.

Use beans to treat the following symptoms: irritability, a tendency toward angry outbursts, tinnitus, temporal headaches, a reddened face and eyes, thirst, constipation characterized by dry stools, and dark-yellow urine.

8 cups of water
1 ounce of peony alba
1 ounce of lycii berries
1/2 ounce of chrysanthemum
8 ounces of chicken or pork (organic, if possible), or 1/2 cup of garbanzo or
     mung beans
1/2 cup of rice
1/2 cup of burdock root (fresh), or 1/4 ounce of dried burdock root
1 cup of carrots
1 cup of beets
1/2 cup of leeks
1/4 cup of celery
6 shiitake mushrooms
1 cup of collard
Fresh cilantro leaves, tumeric, black sesame seeds, salt, and lemon juice (to taste)

When using meat: Cook the pork in six cups of water for 1 hour and 15 minutes, or cook the chicken for 15 minutes. Simmer the peony and burdock (if you're using the dried root) in two cups of water for 15 minutes. Add chrysanthemum and cook the resulting mixture for 15 minutes. Strain this mixture and discard the herbs. Add herb tea and rice to the meat, and cook everything for 30 minutes. Add lycii berries and chopped vegetables (including burdock root, if it's fresh and grated) and cook this mixture for 15 minutes. Finally, add seasonings.

When using beans: Soak the beans for eight hours in six cups of water, then cook them for one hour and 15 minutes. Cook the peony and burdock (if you're using the dried root) in two cups of water for 15 minutes. Add chrysanthemum and cook the resulting mixture for 15 minutes. Strain this mixture and discard the herbs. Add herb tea and rice to the beans, and cook everything for 30 minutes. Add lycii berries and chopped vegetables (including burdock, if it's fresh and grated) and cook this mixture for 15 minutes. Finally, add seasonings.

Congees

A congee is a diluted porridge. Usually, it's made with sweet white or brown rice and water. Congees can also be made with other grains, or a combination of grains, vegetables, beans, animal protein, and herbs. The dish is typically eaten for breakfast; however, weak or chronically ill individuals, or people convalescing from surgery should eat congee at every meal until they recover.

Traditionally, congees are made by cooking one cup of sweet rice with four to six cups of water for about four to six hours, until they reach a porridge-like consistency. Herbs may be added to this mixture and cooked with the rice, at the beginning of the process. Congees are a highly digestible and assimilable food. They are especially good for individuals suffering from weak digestion, poor appetite, gas, bloatedness, abdominal distension, fatigue, and weakness. Congees also act as a tonic for any organ system in the body; their specific effects depend upon the herbs they include. Many of the herbs added to congees may be eaten. The consumption of herbs with congees creates a strong therapeutic action. Honey or raw sugar is sometimes added to sweeten the mixture.

Congee ingredients can be prepared in one of three ways: place them in a crockpot and let them stand overnight; put them in a crockpot—on low—in the morning and let them stand until the end of the day; or prepare them in a glass-covered dish placed in the oven (set at 250 degrees or the lowest oven setting) for eight hours. Congees provide quick but nourishing breakfasts and dinners.

Basic Morning Congee
(*serves four people*)

This congee strengthens digestion, energy, and blood; regulates weight; assists the bowels; and eliminates dampness. It is best eaten with fresh, cooked greens (including kale or collards) and a variety of vegetables.

6 cups of water
6 pitted jujube dates
1/2 ounce of Chinese yam
1/2 cup of rice
1/2 cup of coix or pearled barley

Combine all of the above ingredients and cook them in a glass-covered dish over low heat, for four to six hours; or place them in a crockpot and let them stand for eight to ten hours. If the congee's consistency is too thick for your taste, add some water to thin it. Add honey to the mixture, if desired. This congee can be consumed one to three times a day, as desired.

Sample Congee Recipes

Cold and Flu Congee
(*serves four people*)

This congee relieves colds, flu, and fevers accompanied by slight chills, or without chills.

1/4 ounce of chrysanthemum
1/4 ounce of pueraria
1/4 ounce lily bulb
1/4 ounce of honeysuckle
1 cup of rice

Simmer herbs in two cups of water for 10 minutes, then strain out the dregs. Prepare congee from the resulting liquid and four additional cups of water. Eat this mixture twice a day.

Cold and Flu Congee
(serves four people)

This recipe relieves colds and flu accompanied by chills and a slight fever, or unaccompanied by fever.

6 slices of fresh ginger
3 scallion roots
1/2 cup of rice

Prepare the rice in four cups of water. While the rice is still hot, add scallions and ginger and bring the entire mixture to a boil, cover it, and simmer for five minutes. Eat this mixture on an empty stomach, twice a day. This congee should induce a slight sweat, which will indicate that the condition has improved.

Coughing Congee (Wet Cough)
(serves four people)

This congee alleviates coughing, bronchitis, and the expectoration of lung mucus.

1/2 ounce of almond seed
1/2 ounce of platycodon
1/2 ounce of tangerine peel
1 cup of rice

Prepare tea, with the herbs listed above, in three cups of water. Strain the dregs and use the resulting liquid (with three additional cups of water) to make congee. Consume this congee two to three times a day, as desired.

Coughing Congee (Dry Cough)
(serves four people)

This recipe treats dry coughing accompanied by a dry mouth.

1/4 cup of aduki beans
1/2 ounce of lily bulb
1/4 ounce of apricot seeds
1 cup of rice

Make congee, in six cups of water, with all of the ingredients listed above. Eat the herbs with the congee. Consume this coughing congee two to three times a day, as desired.

Digestive Aid Congee
(serves four people)

This congee alleviates poor digestion, gas, bloatedness, poor appetite, and lethargy.

2 astragalus sticks
2 small codonopsis roots
6 pitted jujube dates
1/4 ounce of Chinese yam
1/4 ounce of tangerine peel
1/4 ounce of hoelen
2 cups of rice
1/2 cup of coix or pearled barley

Cook all of these ingredients together in eight cups of water. Consume all of the herbs except for astragalus and tangerine peel. Eat this congee two to three times a day, as desired.

Digestive Aid Congee
(serves four people)

This recipe regulates diarrhea and fatigue.

1/4 ounce of lotus seeds
1/4 ounce of hoelen
1/8 ounce of dried ginger
1/2 ounce of Chinese yam
1 cup of rice
1/4 cup of coix or pearled barley

Cook these ingredients in six cups of water and eat the resulting congee, with all of the herbs, in the morning.

Constipation Congee
(serves two people)

This congee regulates constipation characterized by coldness and lower-back and knee pain.

1/2 ounce cistanches
4 ounces of lamb
1/2 cup of rice

Simmer the cistanches for 15 minutes in one cup of water. Strain the resulting liquid and cook it with lamb, rice, and three additional cups of water. Eat this congee in the morning on an empty stomach.

Lower-Back Pain Congee
(serves four people)

This congee alleviates lower-back pain, frequent urination, and fatigue.

1/4 ounce of rehmannia
1/4 ounce of *he shou wu*
1/4 ounce of cornus
1/2 ounce of Chinese yam
1 cup of rice

Prepare the herbs as a tea in two cups of water. Strain out the herbs, and keep the Chinese yam in the resulting tea. Cook the tea with rice and add four additional cups water. Consume this congee once or twice a day, as desired.

Sleep Aid Congee
(serves four people)

This recipe treats the symptoms of mental overwork, including insomnia, palpitations, and night sweats.

1/2 ounce of longan berries
1/4 ounce of lotus seeds
1/4 ounce of polygonatum
6 pitted jujube dates
1/4 ounce of hoelen
1 small American ginseng root

1 cup of rice
1/2 cup of coix or pearled barley

Cook all of these ingredients in six cups of water, and eat the resulting congee (with all of the herbs) once or twice a day.

Lowered Immunity Congee
(serves four people)

This recipe relieves lowered immunity, and frequent colds and flu.

2 astragalus sticks
1/4 ounce atractylodis
1/4 ounce siler
1/2 ounce of black fungus (black fungus can be purchased at Chinese herbal pharmacies)
1/2 ounce of black or shiitake mushrooms
1 cup of rice

Prepare the atractylodis and siler as a tea, in one cup of water. Strain the resulting liquid and add it (with the other herbs and rice) to five cups of water. Do not eat the astragalus sticks. Ingest this congee once or twice a day, as desired.

Lowered Immunity and Fatigue Congee
(serves four people)

This congee regulates fatigue, lowered immunity, poor digestion, and poor appetite.

2 astragalus sticks
1 small American ginseng root
2 small codonopsis roots
6 pitted jujube dates
1/4 ounce of Chinese yam
1/4 ounce of hoelen
1/4 ounce of tangerine peel
1/2 cup of rice

Cook these ingredients in eight cups of water. Do not eat the astragalus or tangerine peel. Eat this congee once or twice a day, as desired.

Anemia Congee
(serves six people)

This recipe relieves anemia, weakness, dizziness, blurred vision, short and light menstruation, and amenorrhea.

6 black, pitted jujube dates
2 small codonopsis roots
1/4 ounce of longan berries
1/4 ounce of lycii berries
1/4 ounce of rehmannia
1/4 ounce of cornus
1 cup of rice
1/2 cup coix or pearled barley

Cook these ingredients in six cups of water and eat the resulting congee once or twice a day. Consume all of the herbs but rehmannia.

Infertility Congee
(serves six people)

This congee treats infertility.

1/4 ounce of cornus
1/2 ounce of Chinese yam
1/2 ounce of lycii berries
1/4 ounce of rehmannia
1 small American ginseng root
2 cups of rice

Prepare the cornus and rehmannia as a tea, in one cup of water. Strain the resulting liquid and add it, with the rest of the herbs and two cups of rice, to five cups of water. Consume this congee once or twice a day, as desired.

Energy and Blood Support Congee
(serves four people)

This recipe improves eyesight, nourishes blood, keeps hair its normal color, prevents plaque and cholesterol, regulates the bowels and urinary tract, and supports energy and longevity.

1/2 ounce of he shou wu
1/2 ounce of lycii berries
6 pitted jujube dates
1 cup of rice

Prepare a tea with the *he shou wu*, in one cup of water. Strain the resulting liquid and add it, with the remaining ingredients, to five cups of water. This congee may be eaten daily to promote longevity.

Arthritis and Rheumatism Congee (With Coldness)
(serves four people)

This congee alleviates rheumatic and arthritic pains accompanied by stiffness and cold hands and feet; clear urination; and an aversion to cold.

1 cup of rice
1/4 cup of coix or pearled barley
1/2 ounce of cinnamon-bark powder
1/2 ounce of dried-ginger powder
1/2 ounce of chopped spring onion
Honey (to taste)

Cook the rice with the barley in six cups of water, and add the remaining herbs during the last 15 minutes of preparation. Eat this congee once or twice a day.

Arthritis and Rheumatism Congee (With Heat)
(serves four people)

This recipe treats rheumatic and arthritic pain and stiffness accompanied by inflammation, redness, edema, thirst, and dark-yellow urine.

2 ounces honeysuckle
1/4 cup of red beans
1 cup of coix or pearled barley
1/2 cup of white rice

Cook red beans in six cups of water for one hour and 15 minutes. Add the rice and the barley and cook the resulting mixture for 30 minutes. Place the honeysuckle in a muslin bag, and add it to the congee mixture during the last 15 minutes of preparation. Discard the honeysuckle before eating the congee. Ingest this congee once or twice a day, as desired.

Simple Remedies for Common Ailments

Chinese Herbal Remedies

The herbs listed in each of the following formulas may be powdered and placed in capsules. The standard dosage for each remedy is four capsules three times a day.

Colds, Flu, and Sore Throat

Coldness type: To treat weakness, sweating, chills and slight fever, general achiness, and abdominal pain, decoct 1/2 ounce (each) of cinnamon twigs, peony alba, jujube dates, and fresh ginger, and 1/4 ounce of licorice for ten minutes. The mixture should be prepared in a lid-covered pot. Drink one cup of this tea in the morning and another cup in the evening. Eat a bowl of hot rice or rice cream one-half hour after ingesting the tea.

Heat type: To remedy fever, slight chills, viral infections, acute tonsillitis, coughing, sore throats, general achiness, and the initial stages of measles and mumps, decoct 1 ounce (each) of honeysuckle, forsythia, and gardenia; 1/2 ounce (each) of trichosanthis, platycodon, isatis, and burdock seed; and 1/4 ounce (each) of schizonepeta and licorice from six cups of water to four cups of water. Remove this tea from heat and then add 1/8 ounce of mint. Drink one cup of this tea two to three times a day.

Heat type: To relieve colds, flu, pneumonia, bronchitis, bronchial asthma, measles, fever, lack of sweat, general pain, thirst, coughing, and headaches, decoct 1 ounce (each) of ephedra and apricot seed; 3/4 ounce of cinnamon twig; and 1/4 ounce of licorice from five cups of water down to three cups of water. Add the cinnamon twigs during the last 15 minutes of preparation. Drink one cup of this tea two to three times a day.

Coughing

Coldness type: To alleviate coughing accompanied by white phlegm and feelings of coldness, decoct 1/2 ounce (each) of platycodon, apricot seed, coltsfoot, and licorice from four cups of water down to three cups of water. Drink one cup of this tea two to three times a day.

Heat type: To regulate all types of coughing accompanied by yellow phlegm (including coughing caused by the common cold, pertussis, and bronchitis), decoct 1 ounce (each) of bupleurum and gypsum; 1/2 ounce (each) of platycodon, scute, and morus; and 1/4 ounce (each) of gardenia and licorice. Decoct the gypsum for one-half hour in six cups of water. Add the rest of the herbs and simmer the resulting mixture down to four cups of water. Drink one cup of this tea two to three times a day.

Headaches

Coldness type: To relieve dull and mild headaches, weakness, fatigue, and lack of thirst, decoct 1/2 ounce (each) of ligusticum, angelica, and schizonepeta for ten minutes in two cups of water. Drink one-half cup of this tea three times a day.

Heat type: To treat migraines, headaches, thirst, and the expectoration of yellow mucus, decoct 1/2 ounce (each) of ligusticum and cyperus; 1/4 ounce (each) of angelica, schizonepeta, mint, and siler; and 1/8 ounce (each) of licorice and green tea from four cups of water down to three cups. Add the mint at the end of the decoction process. Drink one cup of this tea two to three times a day.

Nervous Debility, Insomnia, Anxiety

Deficient heat or Qi type: To regulate insomnia, nervous exhaustion, weakness, fatigue, night sweats, nightmares, and palpitations, decoct 1 ounce of zizyphus seeds; 1/2 ounce of hoelen; 1/4 ounce (each) of ligusticum and anemarrhena; and 1/8 ounce of licorice from four cups of water down to three cups. Drink one cup of this tea two to three times a day.

Heat type: To treat insomnia, anxiety, habitual constipation, shoulder stiffness, hypertension, hemorrhoids, and a flushed face, decoct 1/4 ounce (each) of rhubarb, scute, and coptis from two cups water down to one cup. Drink one-half cup of this tea twice a day.

General Fatigue

Coldness type: To relieve anemia, fatigue, loss of weight, and menstrual irregularity, decoct 1/4 ounce (each) of *dang gui*, cooked rehmannia, ligusticum, peony, hoelen, atractylodis, ginseng, and ginger; and 1/8 ounce of licorice from four cups of water down to three cups. Drink one cup of this tea two to three times a day.

Heat type: To remedy fatigue, sensations of chest and abdominal pressure, bloating, belching, nausea, and indigestion characterized by a lack of appetite, decoct 1/4 ounce (each) of ligusticum, gardenia, *shen qu*, cyperus, and *fu ling*; and 1/8 ounce (each) of American ginseng and rhubarb from four cups of water down to three cups. Drink one cup of this tea twice a day.

Gynecological

Coldness type: To alleviate menstrual irregularity, difficult menstruation, weakness, fatigue, lower-back pain, prolonged menstrual flow, anemia, and pallor, decoct 1/2 ounce (each) of peony, hoelen, atractylodis, and alisma; and 1/4 ounce of *dang gui* and ligusticum from six cups of water down to four cups. Drink one cup of this tea two to three times a day.

Heat type: To remedy menstrual irregularity, dysmenorrhea, endometriosis, abnormal menstruation or hemorrhaging, headaches, hypertension, and acute cramping of the lower abdomen, decoct 3/4 ounce of persica, 1/2 ounce of cinnamon twig, 1/4 ounce of rhubarb, and 1/8 ounce of licorice from four cups of water down to three cups. Drink one cup of this tea two to three times a day.

Arthritis and Rheumatism

Coldness type: To remedy arthritis and rheumatism, decoct 1/2 ounce (each) of *dang gui*, cinnamon twigs, peony, and jujube; 1/4 ounce (each) of clematis and licorice; and 1/8 ounce of asarum from six cups of water down to four cups. Add the cinnamon twigs during the last ten minutes of preparation. Drink one cup of this tea two to three times a day.

Heat type: To relieve arthritis characterized by swelling and pain, decoct 1/4 ounce (each) of *dang gui*, anemarrhena, pueraria, atractylodis, alisma, scute, siler, and ginseng; and 1/8 ounce of licorice from four cups of water down to three cups of water. Drink one cup two to three times a day.

Digestive Disturbances

Coldness type: To treat gas, bloatedness, diarrhea or loose stools, fatigue, and poor appetite, decoct 1/3 ounce (each) of codonopsis, atractylodis, and hoelen; 1/4 ounce (each) of ginger, citrus peel, and jujube dates; and 1/8 ounce of licorice from four cups of water down to two cups of water. Drink one cup two to three times a day.

Heat type: To remedy acid regurgitation, abdominal distension and pain, belching, and diarrhea, decoct 1.5 ounces of hawthorn; 3/4 ounce of hoelen; 1/2 ounce of *shen qu*; and 1/4 ounce (each) of citrus peels, radish, and forsythia from six cups of water down to four cups of water. Drink one cup two to three times a day.

Chinese Herbal Patent Remedies

The following is a general outline of diseases and the bulk herbs or patents to use:

SYMPTOMS	REMEDIES
Colds and Flu These are two of the best cold remedies; they are especially effective in the treatment of head colds and sore throats.	*Yin Chiao* Tablets *Ganmaoling*
This patent regulates flu accompanied by high fever and headaches.	*Zhong Gan Ling*
These treatments alleviate stomach flu.	*Huo Hsiang Cheng Chi Pien* Pill Curing
This patent alleviates headaches accompanied by chills, sensations of cold, nasal congestion, sinusitis, or rhinitis.	*Chuan Xiong Chao Tiao Wan*
Coughing This tea relieves dry coughing.	*Lo Han Kuo* Tea
These treatments alleviate heat and coughing accompanied by sticky, yellow phlegm.	Pulmonary Tonic Pills Pinellia Expectorant Pills (*Qing Qi Hua Tan Wan*) Natural Herb Loquat-Flavored Syrup
These pills treat bronchitis.	Bronchitis Pills (Compound)

These pills remedy bronchitis accompanied by lower-back pain and frequent urination.	*Ping Chuan* Pills
These pills regulate acute and chronic bronchitis, and asthma accompanied by coldness.	*Hsiao Keh Chuan* Pills
This patent alleviates sore throats and the expectoration of sticky, yellow phlegm.	*Ching Fei Yi Huo Pien*
This treatment relieves the expectoration of phlegm accompanied by nausea, and chest and abdominal fullness.	*Erh Chen Wan*
This patent treats coughing accompanied by nasal congestion.	*Bi Yan Pian*
These tablets eliminate coughing accompanied by poor digestion or lack of appetite, and loose stools.	*Liu Jun Zi* Tablets

Headaches

These treatments regulate headaches accompanied by fever.	*Yin Chiao* Tablets *Zhong Gan Ling*
This patent relieves headaches accompanied by allergies or sinusitis.	*Bi Yan Pian*
This treatment alleviates headaches and indigestion.	Pill Curing

This patent remedies headaches accompanied by muscle tension or spasms.	*Hsiao Yao Wan*
This treatment relieves headaches accompanied by chills.	*Chuan Xiong Chao Tiao Wan*
This patent regulates migraine pain.	Corydalis *Yanhusus* Analgesic Tablets
This treatment eliminates migraines accompanied by arthritic pain; and arm, leg, or face paralysis.	*Tian Ma Wan*

Allergies or Sinus Infections

These patents alleviate hay fever, and sinusitis accompanied by postnasal drip.	*Bi Yan Pian* *Pe Min Kan Wan*
These pills treat hay fever, allergies, or sinus infections accompanied by thick, sticky, and yellow mucus.	Pinellia Expectorant Pills (*Qing Qi Hua Tan Wan*)
This treatment regulates headache accompanied by sinusitis or rhinitis.	*Chuan Xiong Chao Tiao Wan*

Sore Throats, Mouth Disorders, and Ear Problems

This patent treats sore throats, swollen gums, toothaches, nosebleeds, ear infections, and hives.	*Huang Lien Shang Ching Pien*

These pills alleviate acute throat inflammation, swollen glands, measles, and abscesses.	*Chuan Xin Lian* (Antiphlogistic Pills)
These pills relieve laryngitis, acute tonsillitis, and mumps.	Laryngitis Pills
This patent eliminates mouth sores, mouth ulcers, and toothaches.	*Xi Gua Shuang*
This powder spray soothes sore throats.	Superior Sore Throat Powder Spray
These pills treat sore throats, fever blisters on the mouth, red and burning eyes, and headaches.	*Lung Tan Xie Gan* Pills
These pills regulate tinnitus, high blood pressure, insomnia, thirst, and eye irritation.	*Tso-Tzu Otic* Pills

Eyes

This patent relieves reddened, itching, and swollen eyes; and photophobia.	*Ming Mu Shang Ching Pien*
These pills improve vision and alleviate pressure behind eyes, blurriness, cataracts, and dry eyes.	Dendrobrum Moniliforme Night Sight Pills
These pills treat reddened and burning eyes, and headaches.	*Lung Tan Xie Gan* Pills

Genitourinary

This patent eliminates acute vaginitis, and cystitis caused by yeast.

Yudai Wan

This treatment alleviates acute cystitis, prostatitis, and urethritis.

Lung Tan Xie Gan Pills

This patent remedies acute cystitis or vaginitis accompanied by thirst, hot flashes, night sweats, and insomnia.

Eight-Flavor Tea

These pills treat chronic vaginitis.

Chien Chin Chih Tai Wan

This treatment regulates chronic urethritis; and urinary calculi in the kidney, bladder, or ureters.

Specific Drug Passwan

This patent alleviates chronic prostatitis.

Kai Kit Wan

Gynecological Conditions

This patent treats premenstrual syndrome, menstrual irregularity, and depression.

Hsiao Yao Wan

These treatments regulate menstrual irregularity, fatigue, poor appetite, menstrual cramps, and premenstrual syndrome.

Wu Chi Pai Feng Wan
(White Phoenix Pills)
Pai Feng Wan

These tablets treat menstrual irregularity and excessive uterine bleeding.

Butiao Tablets

This patent alleviates menstrual irregularity, fatigue, anemia, the emission of pale blood, palpitations, poor memory, dizziness, and amenorrhea.	*Tang Kwe Gin*
These pills relieve night sweats, hot flashes, and dizziness.	Placenta Compound Restorative Pills (*He Che Da Zao Wan*)
This treatment alleviates uterine bleeding, chronic miscarriage, and uterine or bladder prolapse.	Central *Qi* Pills (*Bu Zhong Yi Qi Wan*)
This tea treats impotence, infertility, and coldness.	Golden Book Tea
This tea regulates light or irregular menses, dizziness, poor memory, a pale face, and fatigue.	Eight-Treasure Tea
This patent calms restless fetal movement, and prevents impending miscarriage.	*An Tai Wan*
This treatment prevents impending miscarriage during the first trimester of pregnancy.	*Shih San Tai Pao Wan*
This patent regulates uterine bleeding, irregular or heavy menses, night sweats, insomnia, and palpitations.	*Gui Pi Wan*

Hemorrhoids
This patent relieves hemorrhoidal pain, itching, burning, and bleeding.	Fargelin (For Piles)

This treatment eliminates hemor-rhoidal bleeding.

Yunnan Paiyao

Digestive Disorders
These pills treat poor digestion, bloating, the elimination of loose stools, and loss of appetite.

Ginseng Stomachic Pills
(*Ren Shen Jian Pi Wan*)

These tablets alleviate poor diges-tion, the elimination of loose stools, chronic diarrhea, acid regurgitation, and nausea.

Liu Jun Zi Tablets

This patent regulates poor diges-tion and absorption of food.

Ginseng Royal-Jelly Vials

These pills remedy poor digestion, diarrhea, vomiting or nausea, the elimination of clear urine, and cold hands or feet.

Carmichaeli Tea Pills
(*Fu Zi Li Zhong Wan*)

This treatment eliminates gas, hiccups, belching, the elimina-tion of loose or erratic stools, nausea, and regurgitation.

Shu Kan Wan (condensed)

This patent treats bloating, hic-cups, poor appetite, food allergies, premenstrual syndrome, and depression.

Hsiao Yao Wan
(Bupleurum Sedative Pills)

These pills relieve bloating, gas, the elimination of erratic stools, chronic diarrhea, low energy, and organ or anal prolapse.

Central *Qi* Pills
(*Bu Zhong Yi Qi Wan*)

This patent remedies diarrhea, food congestion, nausea, vomiting, the elimination of pasty stools, and flatulence.	*Huo Hsiang Cheng Chi Pien*
This treatment alleviates food congestion or poisoning, overeating, acute diarrhea, mild constipation, and motion sickness.	Pill Curing
This patent relieves abdominal cramping or bloating, poor appetite, diarrhea, nausea, and pain.	*Ping Wei Pian*
These pills eliminate constipation, food congestion, foul-smelling belches and breath, and hypoacidity.	*Mu Xiang Shun Qi Wan* (Aplotaxis Carminative Pills)
This treatment regulates chronic constipation.	*Fructus Persica* Compound Pills
This formula treats duodenal and gastric ulcers unaccompanied by bleeding, hyperacidity, and gastritis.	*Sai Mei An* (Internal Formula)
Use this patent, in addition to the patent listed immediately above, to treat the symptoms listed immediately above when they are accompanied by bleeding.	*Yunnan Paiyao*
Use this patent to alleviate digestive disorders accompanied by pain and bleeding, including duodenal and gastric ulcers.	*Wei Te Ling*

Liver and Gallbladder Disorders These tablets alleviate gallstones.	Lidan Tablets
This treatment remedies jaundice, hepatitis, and gallstones.	*Li Gan Pian*
These pills regulate acute and chronic hepatitis accompanied by jaundice.	*Ji Gu Cao* pill
Heart Disorders This patent regulates angina, palpitations, cholesterol levels, and the production of lipids.	*Danshen* Tabletco
This treatment relieves the following stroke symptoms: paralysis and impaired speech.	*Ren Shen Zai Zao Wan*
This patent treats palpitations; angina; heart disorders accompanied by face, arm, or leg paralysis; and migraine pain.	*Tian Ma Wan*
Skin Disorders These pills remedy acne, furuncles, itching, rashes, and hives.	Margarite Acne Pills
These patents relieve abscesses, carbuncles, and rashes.	*Lien Chiao Pai Tu Pien* *Chuan Xin Lian*
These patents alleviate hives and itching.	Margarite Acne Pills *Huang Lien Shang Ching Pien*
This treatment regulates boils, and nose and mouth sores.	*Ching Fei Yi Huo Pian*

Arthritis and Rheumatism

This patent treats lower-back pain and sciatica.

Specific Lumbaglin

This treatment remedies lower-back and knee pain accompanied by sensations of coldness.

Du Huo Jisheng Wan

This patent alleviates rheumatism, stiff joints, and numbness.

Xiao Huo Luo Dan

This treatment relieves arthritis and rheumatism accompanied by stiff joints, numbness, sciatica, and sensations of coldness.

Feng Shih Hsiao Tung Wan

This patent regulates arthritis and rheumatism accompanied by coldness; face, arm, or leg paralysis; and migraine pain.

Tian Ma Wan

Insomnia

This patent treats difficulty in falling asleep, mental agitation or exhaustion, excess dreaming, and poor memory.

An Mien Pien

This treatment regulates difficulty in falling asleep, anxiety, palpitations, and dizziness.

Ding Xin Wan

This patent relieves difficulty in staying asleep, nightmares, night sweats, palpitations, and fatigue.

Shen Ching Shuai Jao Wan

This treatment eliminates vivid dreaming, anxiety, and palpitations.	Emperor's Tea (*Tian Wang Bu Xin Wan*)
This patent remedies excessive dreaming, palpitations, poor memory, restlessness, and dizziness.	*An Sheng Bu Xin Wan*
This treatment remedies palpitations, restless dreaming, nightmares, night sweats, and dizziness.	*Gui Pi Wan*

Hypertension

These tablets regulate hypertension accompanied by sensations of coldness, lower-back pain, fatigue, frequent urination, and palpitations.	Compound Cortex Eucommia Tablets (*Fu Fang Du Zhong Pian*)
This patent relieves hypertension accompanied by sensations of heat, tinnitus (ear ringing), constipation, thirst, expectoration of yellow phlegm, and a flushed face.	Hypertension Repressing Tablets (*Jiang Ya Ping Pian*)
This treatment regulates hypertension accompanied by tinnitus, insomnia, sore throats, eye irritation and pressure, and headaches.	*Tso-Tzu Otic* Pills

Energy Tonics

These pills treat lowered energy accompanied by organ or anal prolapse and poor digestion.	Central *Qi* Pills (*Bu Zhong Yi Qi Wan*)
These patents relieve lowered energy characterized by a pale face, weakness, anemia, hypoglycemia, and low appetite.	Eight-Treasure Tea *Tang Kwe Gin*

This tea regulates lowered energy accompanied by sensations of coldness, lower-back aches, and the elimination of undigested food.	Golden Book Tea (Sexoton Pills)
These pills remedy general weakness and promote longevity.	Yang Rong Wan (Ginseng Tonic Pills)
This tea treats lowered energy accompanied by sore throats, weakness, mild night sweats, dizziness, and impotence.	Six Flavor Tea (*Liu Wei Di Huang Wan*)
This patent alleviates fatigue accompanied by palpitations, insomnia, dizziness, and uterine bleeding.	Gui Pi Wan

Pediatric Disorders

This treatment relieves fever, coughing, measles, colds, and the expectoration of mucus.	Hui Chun Tan
These pills remedy fever, coughing, teething, and diarrhea.	Bo Ying Pills
This patent alleviates sore throats, mouth sores, swollen gums, reddened eyes, and constipation.	Tao Chih Pien (For Babies)

Trauma

This treatment relieves pain caused by sprains, fractures, and hemorrhages; shock; and external bleeding.	Yunnan Paiyao
This liniment treats bruising, ligament and muscle tears, fractures, and sprains.	Zheng Gu Shui

Understanding Disease

The Five Elements

The Five Elements provide a theoretical framework that defines the relationship between nature and the human body. This system—developed approximately 2,500 years ago—describes the influence of factors such as emotions, seasons, climate, food, color, and sound on the organs of the body. The Five Elements are wood, fire, metal, earth, and water. Wood represents the liver and gallbladder; fire includes the heart and small intestine; earth encompasses the spleen and stomach; metal represents the lungs and large intestine; and water includes the kidneys and urinary bladder.

Each of the Five Elements corresponds to a component of nature; these corollary components describe the Element and facilitate diagnosis and treatment. The Five Elements and their corresponding components are listed on the next page.

Element	Wood	Fire	Earth	Metal	Water
Yin organs	liver	heart	spleen	lung	kidney
Yang organs	gallbladder	small intestine	stomach	large intestine	urinary bladder
Opens to	eyes	tongue	mouth	nose	ears
Sense	sight	speech	taste	smell	hearing
Fluids	tears, bile	sweat, blood	lymph, saliva	mucus	spinal, sexual
Rules	tendons	pulse	muscles	skin, body hair	bones, head hair
Emotions	anger	overex- citement	melancholy, worry	grief	fear
Sounds	shouting	laughter	song	sobbing	groaning
Colors	green	red	yellow	white	black, dark blue
Tastes	sour	bitter	sweet	pungent	salty
Activities	looking	walking	sitting	reclining	standing
Energies	wind	heat	dampness	dryness	cold
Seasons	spring	summer	Indian summer	autumn	winter
Directions	east	south	center	west	north
Injurious influences	wind	heat	moisture	dryness	cold
External aspects	nails	complexion	lips	body hair	head hair, anus
Spiritual influences	Ethereal Soul	Spirit (Shen)	Thought	Corporeal Soul	Will
Grains	wheat	corn	millet	rice	beans
Animals	chicken	lamb	cow	horse	pig
Fruits	plums	apricots	dates	peaches	chestnuts

Organs correspond to the Five Elements through diagnosis, therapy, and constitution. Following is an example of the correlation between one Element and its related organs: the Fire Element encompasses its *yin* organ (the heart) and its *yang* organ (the small intestine). The heart opens to the tongue, so speech problems are indicative of a heart imbalance. Fire (or heat) causes movement, while lack of fire results in an absence or dysfunction of proper or appropriate movement. People who dislike speaking or who stutter display a heart-energy weakness, while individuals who talk incessantly have a heart-energy excess. Either of these conditions is indicative of a heart, or Fire Element, imbalance.

Additionally, walking helps the heart—since it circulates blood—and an individual with poor circulation benefits from walking. This form of exercise, in moderation, can also be therapeutic for people with weakened hearts. However, excessive walking can further weaken the heart and should be avoided by those individuals with a Fire Element imbalance. Excessive heat, caused by overexertion or climatic influence, injures the heart. Eating foods with a bitter taste helps eliminate excessive heat in the heart.

The energy of the Fire Element, as it pertains to constitution, tends towards interpersonal communication and relationships. An individual with a fire-type constitution is predisposed to overexcitement or indulgence, since s/he often likes to be in the midst of a group, talking, laughing, and having a good time. People with fire-type constitutions generally have red cheeks; shiny eyes; positive, happy personalities; and sharp minds.

The Five Element System describes our bodily need to maintain balance through cravings and desires. Individuals lacking in earth energy, for instance, may experience exceptional cravings for sweets. The ingestion of a moderate amount of balanced carbohydrates and proteins helps satisfy these cravings and remedies spleen deficiencies, while the consumption of a concentrated amount of strong, sweet-tasting foods overstimulates the spleen and causes further cravings. Similarly, a temperate intake of sea salt, miso, tamari, and seaweeds helps strengthen the kidneys (or Water Element), while excessive consumption of these foods injures and weakens them.

Each of the Five Elements embodies a particular energy or power. Wood signifies birth, creativity, and expression; fire indicates impulse, consciousness, Spirit, and the mental processes; earth encompasses centeredness, nourishment, and the ability to concentrate; metal represents elimination, letting go, regulation, and energy-conduction throughout the body; and water designates willpower, essential power, inherited constitution, and fluidity. All of these qualities are active when their corollary organs are in balance. When their corollary organs are in a state of excess, these powers are overstimulated; conversely, if a particular organ is in a state of deficiency, its corresponding Element will be suppressed.

You can identify people's Five-Element imbalances by observing how they walk or sit; their taste and color preferences; tone of voice; personality type; and so on. Our identities—how we act, feel, and think—portray our predominant constitutional Element and its imbalances.

Individuals who worry about money; express attitudes of insufficiency and inadequacy; need to sit and cannot stand for very long; have a light and low groaning tone to their everyday voice; and a darkish color to the skin (especially under the eyes) have a water imbalance. People with water imbalances tend to have inherited weaknesses; lack willpower; lack power or strength; experience lower-back and joint aches; and tend towards fatigue. Herbs with a salty taste, such as seaweeds, help strengthen the Water Element.

Timid or repressed people, with little tendency towards self-expression, or individuals who are overly creative have a wood imbalance. Either version of this imbalance can lead to feelings of frustration, anger, moodiness, and depression. Individuals suffering from wood imbalances generally manifest a shouting tone of voice; a greenish cast to their skin; inflexibility in body or mind; ridged and yellow nails; or reddened, tearing eyes. Herbs with a sour taste, like schisandra, can assist the liver function.

Fire imbalances are indicated by the presence of an inappropriately happy or over-indulgent party mood; or a marked absence of happiness and joy. This imbalance may also cause speech difficulties, excessive sweating, overexcitement, or palpitations. A fire, or heart, imbalance may cause a variety of psychological problems, all of which affect one's ability to relate to the external world. These problems include neurosis and schizophrenia. Herbs with a bitter taste, such as coptis, strengthen the Fire Element.

An earth imbalance manifests itself in problems of assimilation, whether of food, drink, or (on a more subtle level) ideas and concepts. In this imbalance, individuals tend to display a lack of centeredness and grounding; the need to seek personal support from others; a yellowish pallor; an overly sweet manner of expression; a singsong voice; or a total absence of vocal inflection.

Individual's with an earth imbalance may also crave sweets, have dry or red lips, and tend toward edema. Herbs with a sweet flavor—like licorice or jujube dates—enhance the Earth Element.

A metal imbalance causes inability to relinquish the past, either psychologically or physically (as shown in constipation). Individuals with this imbalance generally display a whining or sobbing tone to their voice; a whitish pallor; a tendency toward the expectoration of mucus; physical weakness; lung problems; sinus congestion; and coughing. Herbs with a pungent taste—like ginger—assist the Metal Element.

The Five Elements are also known as the Five Phases, because each Element has a dynamic interrelationship with other Elements. These relationships are incorporated into two main cycles: the *Shen* cycle and the *Ko* cycle. A recognition of these interrelationships is critical to the diagnosis of constitutional types, and acts as a guide to a healthy way of life. This system shows us how an imbalance in one organ process influences an imbalance in all the other organs, and how we can harmonize the organs to create balance in our lives.

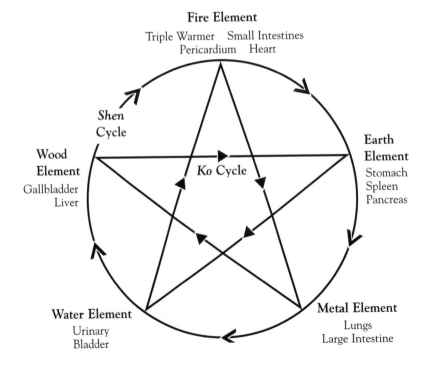

Fire Element
Triple Warmer   Small Intestines
Pericardium   Heart

Shen Cycle

Wood Element
Gallbladder
Liver

Ko Cycle

Earth Element
Stomach
Spleen
Pancreas

Water Element
Urinary
Bladder

Metal Element
Lungs
Large Intestine

The *Shen* cycle moves clockwise; it consists of an engendering, supportive, or nurturing movement. Within this cycle, fire creates ash, which engenders earth; earth harbors metal; melted metal turns into a liquid, which creates fluidity; water nourishes the growth of the plant kingdom, which engenders wood; and finally, burning wood feeds fire. This engendering cycle is described as a parent-child relationship; fire is the parent of earth, earth is the parent of metal, and so forth. Therefore, the parent Element is responsible for nurturing its child, or the Element that it engenders.

The *Ko* cycle is sometimes called the controlling cycle. According to this model, wood controls earth by pushing up soil during its growth; earth controls water by damming it; water controls fire by extinguishing it; fire controls metal by melting it; and metal controls wood by breaking it. Interrelations within the controlling cycle are called grandparent-grandchild relationships; they reflect the role of grandparents, with their control over grandchildren's behavior, as the protectors of custom and tradition in traditional Chinese society. As such, wood is the grandparent of earth, earth is the grandparent of water, and so forth. The grandparent Element controls, or keeps in check, its grandchild organ.

Within each Element, closely related *yin* and *yang* organs follow the husband-wife law. *Yang* organs store *qi*, blood, and fluids; while *yin* organs transform *qi*, blood, and fluids. *Yin* organs are vital to life, and are considered to be the more important (or dominant) set of organs. This law states that aid given to one interrelated organ benefits its partner, and that to harm one interrelated organ is to harm the other. The stomach is husband to the spleen; the large intestine is husband to the lungs; the kidneys are wife to the urinary bladder; the liver is wife to the gallbladder; and the small intestine is husband to the heart.

Treating the stomach (the husband) assists assimilation, as represented by the spleen (the wife); and treating the kidneys (the wife) helps the bladder (the husband) to retain urine, and so forth. On the other hand, a depletion of the lungs (the wife) can lead to a depletion of the large intestine (the husband). This depletion causes constipation resulting from lack of energy.

Health reflects a dynamic interaction between all Five Elements. In sickness, an imbalance in one Element causes an imbalance in that Element's parent, child, grandparent, or grandchild corollaries, as explained through the *Shen* or *Ko* cycles. These imbalances manifest themselves on physical, mental, and emotional levels.

For example: If wood (the grandparent) is in excess, it overcontrols earth (the grandchild). This overcontrol causes nausea, indigestion, gas, acid belching, and alternating constipation and diarrhea. If earth (the grandparent) overdominates water (the grandchild), urinary problems may result. If water (the grandparent) overcontrols fire (the grandchild), it may lead to edema and water retention-related heart problems.

When earth (the parent) is in excess, it causes an imbalance in metal (the child), resulting in digestive problems characterized by the presence of lung or sinus mucus. If water (the parent) is weakened by excessive standing, overactivity, lack of rest, excessive sexual activity, or overindulgence in sugar, alcohol, or caffeine, it cannot nourish wood (the child). This imbalance results in a tight neck and shoulders; headaches or migraines; spasmodic side or rib pains; and a marked tendency towards anger, irritability, or depression.

The Five Elements also direct guidance and counseling. We can help a person who experiences sadness or grief (metal emotions) by giving them sympathy. This process uses the Earth Element (the mother) to nourish the Metal Element (the child). Similarly, when joy and laughter help a person overcome grief and sadness, it is as a result of fire (the grandparent) controlling metal (the grandchild).

Anger (the emotion of wood) is increased by the water emotion of fear, but controlled by the metal emotion of sadness or grief. Fear (the emotion of water) is lessened by the emotion of earth, which includes feelings of pleasure, comfort, and a heightened sense of one's center. Anger can activate and motivate a person steeped in nostalgia and melancholy (earth emotions), and lead to a deepened sense of joy and happiness (fire emotions) when causative issues are resolved.

Although the Five Element system aids us in identification and comprehension of underlying constitutions, this knowledge (in and of itself) does not provide enough information to effectively treat acute colds, flu, skin conditions, or digestive disorders. Generally, when we identify Five Element correlations, we find that all Five Element indications are present in everyone. As such, the key to diagnosis is recognizing primary imbalances.

While Five Element analysis offers a more fundamental understanding of the causes of disease, other Traditional Chinese Medicine systems (such as Eight Principles) afford a more direct treatment strategy. Five Element imbalances tend to remain even after an original complaint is resolved. We all exhibit a predominance or deficiency of one Element or another.

The Five Element system is like a "user's guide" to the specific needs and requirements of the individual body. By learning to recognize our tendencies and limitations according to the Five Element system, we are better able to utilize the various aspects of this system to create greater harmony and well-being in our lives. The dominant principle of the Five Element system is that energy should continue to flow with integrity, grace, compassion, and awareness. It is with this end in mind that acupuncture, dietary medicine, and herbal medicine are employed.

Causes of Disease

In Traditional Chinese Medicine (TCM), there are three major causes of disease: external factors; emotional issues; and miscellaneous causes of disease, including an imbalanced lifestyle.

External Factors

External causes of disease are attributed to the Six Pernicious Influences. These influences are environmental factors that, when we are overexposed to them, can invade the body and cause disease.

Wind

Like meteorological wind, pathogenic wind causes movement, either externally or internally. It migrates to different parts of the body and changes the direction, location, and intensity of various symptoms. Pathogenic wind leads to the following symptoms: spasms; twitches; dizziness; muscle rigidity; deviations of the eye and mouth, as found in Bell's palsy; a stiff or rigid neck and shoulders; tremors; convulsions; vertigo; and the sudden onset of colds, chills, fever, stuffy nose, and headache.

Wind generally accompanies cold or heat factors, termed wind-chill or wind-heat. Wind-chill manifests itself in the sudden onset of slight fever accompanied by strong chills; aversion to wind and cold; body aches; headaches; an itchy or slight sore throat; the expectoration of clear-to-white phlegm; and lack of sweating. Wind-heat's symptoms include the sudden onset of high fever accompanied by slight chills; aversion to wind and heat; a swollen, sore throat; the expectoration of yellow phlegm; and sweating.

Cold
Cold causes sensations of coldness, and a slowing of circulation and all metabolic functions. Symptoms include coldness, clear-to-white bodily secretions, chills, body aches, poor circulation, frequent and copious urination, the elimination of loose stools or diarrhea, the appearance of undigested food in the stools, poor digestion, and a lack of appetite. Cold can appear with both wind and dampness.

Heat
Pathogenic heat causes thirst; dryness; constipation; hemorrhaging; bloody vomit, urine, stools, noses, or mucus; burning sensations; strong odors; sticky or thick, yellow bodily excretions; restlessness; irritability; scant, dark-yellow urination; swollen, red, and painful eyes or gums; and red skin eruptions. Heat can appear with wind or dampness.

Dryness
Dryness is characterized by dehydration. Dehydration is caused by heat, or by blood or *yin* deficiencies. Dryness manifests itself in the following symptoms: extreme thirst; dry skin, hair, mouth, lips, nose, or throat; dry coughing; and constipation.

Dampness
Dampness manifests itself in the presence of excessive bodily fluids. Its symptoms include heaviness; sluggishness; turbid, sluggish, sinking, viscous, copious, slimy, cloudy, or sticky secretions; excessive leukorrhea; oozing, purulent skin eruptions; lassitude; edema; abdominal distension; chest fullness; nausea; and aching, heavy, stiff, and sore joints.

Dampness appears with either heat or coldness. In both cases, signs of dampness include heaviness; sluggishness; distension; chest fullness; nausea;

and aching, heavy, stiff joints. When dampness accompanies heat, secretions or excretions are thick, sticky, and yellow. Damp-cold secretions or excretions are clear-to-white, copious, and runny.

Summer Heat

Summer Heat is another term for heatstroke. This is a condition of extreme, acute heat, which causes the following symptoms: sudden, very high fever; heavy sweating; extreme thirst; nausea; an upset and flushed face; and exhaustion. Summer Heat can lead to loss of consciousness.

The Seven Emotions

TCM teaches that internal diseases are often caused by the Seven Emotions, which include: joy, sadness, anger, grief, melancholy, fear and fright. The physiological relationship between the emotions and the immune system is of tremendous importance. Overexpression or repression of emotions tends to make us vulnerable to chronic disease, and chronic disease makes us vulnerable to overexpression or repression of emotions.

Overexpression of a particular emotion will, in time, injure the organ to which the emotion is related. Conversely, an imbalanced organ system can cause an intensified experience of its related emotion. The resolution of emotional issues helps heal organs and the body. Likewise, treatment of the body lessens the expression or experience of particular emotions.

A person who is frequently irritable, angry, frustrated, or depressed may cause their liver to congest, or create more heat in the liver. This process, in turn, can lead to the following symptoms: a reddened face and eyes; tinnitus; dizziness; migraines; a tight neck and shoulders; disturbed sleep; constipation; premenstrual syndrome; irregular or painful menstruation; and nausea, vomiting, and other digestive difficulties. Conversely, a person who suffers from these symptoms (as caused by a diet excessive in fats, alcohol, or caffeine; a stressful lifestyle; and long-term, unexpressed emotions) may begin to express irritability, frustration, depression and anger for "no apparent reason."

If this person works on the appropriate expression and release of frustration, irritability, and anger (through writing, pounding pillows, creativity, movement, etc.), his or her liver will decongest and liver heat will dissipate. Similarly, the use of herbs (such as dandelion and chicory), the alteration of lifestyle habits, and a change in diet will clear stagnation and heat in the liver, and the individual in question will be less prone to angry outbursts or depression.

Joy
Within the framework of the Seven Emotions, joy is characterized by overexcitability. This condition injures the heart and can lead to insomnia, anxiety, muddled thinking, inappropriate crying or laughter, fits, hysteria, and insanity.

Anger
Resentment, frustration, irritability, rage, indignation, bitterness, animosity, and anger injure the liver and cause headaches, tinnitus, dizziness, blurred vision, mental confusion, bloody vomit, hypertension, premenstrual syndrome, depression, swollen breasts prior to periods, irregular or painful periods, and digestive upset.

Sadness
Sadness affects both the lungs and heart and results in breathlessness, depression or crying, fatigue, amenorrhea, shortness of breath, lowered resistance to colds and flu, palpitations, dizziness, insomnia, and anxiety.

Melancholy
Melancholy is also known as pensiveness or obsessiveness. It disrupts the functions of the spleen and causes fatigue, loss of appetite, dampness, weak digestion, abdominal distension, loose stools, anemia, and lowered immunity.

Grief
Grief impairs the lungs and leads to shortness of breath, expectoration of mucus, sweating, fatigue, coughing, allergies, asthma, pneumonia, bronchitis, emphysema and other lung complaints, anxiety, and susceptibility to colds and flu.

Fear
Insecurity, paranoia, and fear injure the kidneys and adrenals and cause bedwetting, frequent urination, urinary incontinence, lower-back and knee pains, ear infections, infertility, lowered libido, premature signs of age, and lowered immunity.

Fright

Fright injures both the kidneys and the heart and results in palpitations, breathlessness, insomnia, dizziness, tinnitus, night sweats, and chronic fatigue.

In TCM, treatment of excessively expressed or repressed emotions (the vices) occurs through a focus on the vices' corresponding emotional virtues. In ancient times, physicians encouraged their patients to change vices into virtues. This process was called "culturing the virtue." These physicians used one emotion to overcome another. Taoism, the philosophy underlying Traditional Chinese Medicine, also focused on personality alteration.

The following chart indicates the relationship between particular organs and specific emotions.

ORGAN	VICE	VIRTUE
liver	anger, frustration	benevolence, forgiveness, esteem, respect
heart	overexcitement, over achievement	compassion, care of one's self
lungs	grief, sadness	conscientiousness, feeling good about one's self
spleen	obsession, overthinking	empathy, centeredness
kidneys	fear, paranoia, worry	courage, wisdom

Organs may also be healed through the provision of their essential needs. These needs, as related to specific organs, are listed below.

- liver: relaxation, peace, herbs
- heart: love, joy, beauty
- lungs: confidence, time and space
- spleen: nurturance, nutrition
- kidneys: quiet, meditation, rest, sleep, consumption of water

Miscellaneous Causes of Disease

Improper diet, trauma, animal or insect bites, imbalanced lifestyle, parasites, toxins, weak constitution, malnutrition, and food poisoning also cause disease.

Lifestyle and diet are the most important of these factors. Factors that lead to an imbalanced lifestyle include excessive sexual, physical, and mental activity; inactivity; inadequate sleep; and lack of exercise. Issues of diet are covered in the chapter entitled "Chinese Herbal Diet," on page 129. Lifestyle habits are discussed below.

Lifestyle Habits

Sexuality

Sexual activity (known traditionally by the Chinese as "affairs of the bedroom") in excess is deleterious to health, because it depletes kidney Essence. The results of this depletion include lower-back pain, dizziness, low energy, premature signs of age, dental problems, tinnitus, loss of hearing, and loss of eyesight. Excessive sexual activity, within this framework, refers specifically to ejaculation and orgasm; periodic sexual stimulation unaccompanied by ejaculation actually promotes youthful vigor. There are a number of ancient treatises on the practice of Taoist sexual yoga, which improves health and longevity.

Physical Activity

Lack of physical activity causes the energy and blood to stagnate. This process, in turn, leads to reduced organ-system functioning. The reduction of organ-system functioning induces fatigue, lowered immunity, poor circulation, dampness, and a hypofunctioning of bodily processes.

In today's society, overactivity is as common a problem as lack of physical activity. We now accomplish within days or hours what would have taken years; this acceleration creates burnout, or deficient heat. Deficient heat results in night sweats, insomnia, exhaustion accompanied by restlessness, a burning sensation in the palms of hands or soles of feet, and lowered immunity. Stress caused by overexertion is a major cause of hypertension, heart disease, and other debilitating ailments.

Energy expended in the accomplishment of daily activities is easily replenished, under normal circumstances, by proper diet and rest. However, continued intense activity (e.g., working for long, hard hours, months, or even years without adequate rest) results in a bodily inability to restore energy. In this case, the body is forced to draw on its Essence reserves, which ultimately creates deficient heat.

Overexertion exists in one of three forms: mental overexertion, physical overexertion, and excessive exercise. Mental overwork encompasses long work hours, often accomplished in a confined space, under unreasonable deadlines and conditions of stress. This state also results in skipped, late, or irregular meals, which further contributes to energy and yin deficiencies. Physical overexertion causes energy depletion, which leads to blood and yin deficiencies. Excessive exercise depletes energy, blood, yin, and Essence.

Various postures and movements benefit or injure specific organs. Sitting, which is associated with the spleen, is beneficial in moderation. In excess, sitting causes poor digestion; poor assimilation; and swelling of the lymph in the abdomen, hips, and thighs. Excessive standing injures the kidneys, which leads to lower-back pain and frequent urination. Excessive walking can deplete the liver. Overreading, or excessive use of the eyes, damages the heart and causes insomnia or restless sleep. Excessive lying down injures the lungs and leads to shortness of breath, accumulation of lung phlegm, and aggravates existing lung conditions (such as bronchitis or asthma).

Other

The body conforms to a specific biorhythm cycle; as such, there are optimal times of day during which to perform specific activities. Refer to the Chinese biorhythm chart, shown below, which lists the appropriate times of day for organ-related activities.

TIME	ORGAN
11 A.M. to 1 P.M.	heart
1 P.M. to 3 P.M.	small intestine
3 P.M. to 5 P.M.	bladder
5 P.M. to 7 P.M.	kidney-adrenals
7 P.M. to 9 P.M.	pericardium
9 P.M. to 11 P.M.	triple warmer
11 P.M. to 1 A.M.	gallbladder

1 A.M. to 3 A.M.	liver
3 A.M. to 5 A.M.	lungs
5 A.M. to 7 A.M.	large intestine
7 A.M. to 9 A.M.	stomach
9 A.M. to 11 A.M.	spleen/pancreas

As stated above, certain activities are appropriate to different times of day. For example, defecation ideally occurs during the period of time optimal for large-intestine activity (between 5 A.M. and 7 A.M.). Also, according to this system, a nutritious breakfast should be consumed between 7 A.M. and 9 A.M., the period best suited to stomach activity. Sleep taken between 11 P.M. and 3 A.M. provides the greatest amount of regeneration, since it is during wood time (11 p.m. to 3 a.m.) that the liver cleans and replenishes the blood.

Similarly, organic imbalances and weaknesses are likely to appear at certain times; as such, the chart above is useful as a diagnostic tool. For example, it is common for individuals with weak kidney energy to grow tired in the late afternoon, during water time (between 3 P.M. and 7 P.M.). Also, people with lung ailments often wake up between 3 A.M. and 5 A.M., have difficulty breathing, and can't go back to sleep.

Glossary: Terms of Traditional Chinese Medicine

Aromatic stomachic: These herbs are aromatic, and assist digestion by moving dampness.

Blood: This substance encompasses the physical blood in the body. It moistens the tissues, muscles, skin, and hair, and nourishes cells and organs.

Blood deficiency: A blood deficiency is a lack of blood, which is generally accompanied by the following symptoms: anemia; dizziness; scant menses (amenorrhea); a thin, emaciated body; the appearance of spots in the visual field; impaired vision; numb arms or legs; dry skin, hair, or eyes; lusterless, pale face and lips; fatigue; and poor memory.

Bodily fluids: see Fluids.

Calmative: This treatment calms the mind and nerves. It is used to heal nervous disorders.

Cold, coldness, and cold signs: These states are a result of lowered metabolism, and are usually characterized by the following symptoms: aversion to cold and craving for heat; clear-to-white bodily secretions; chills; body aches; poor circulation; a pale complexion; lethargy; lack of thirst; lack of sweat; frigidity; impotence; infertility; nighttime urination; frequent and copious urination; the elimination of loose stools (diarrhea); the presence of undigested food in the stools; poor digestion; lack of appetite; low fever accompanied by severe chills; and hypoconditions, including hypothyroidism, hypoadrenalism, and hypoglycemia.

Cools blood: This process is a function of certain herbs that clear heat from the blood. Symptoms of heat in the blood include rashes, nosebleeds, vomiting, expectoration of blood, bloody stools or urine, night fevers, delirium, and hemorrhaging.

Damp, dampness: Damp and dampness are characterized by the presence of excessive bodily fluids. Symptoms of this condition include feelings of heaviness or sluggishness; turbid, sluggish, sinking, viscous, copious, slimy, cloudy, or sticky secretions; excessive leukorrhea; oozing, purulent skin eruptions; lassitude; edema; abdominal distension; chest fullness; nausea; vomiting; loss of appetite; lack of thirst; and aching, heavy, stiff, and sore joints.

Damp heat: This is a condition of both dampness and heat. Its symptomology includes: thick, greasy, yellow secretions and phlegm; jaundice; hepatitis; dysentery; urinary difficulty or pain; furuncles; and eczema.

Deficiency: A deficiency is a condition of weakness; it consists of a lack of qi, blood, fluids, *yin, yang*, or Essence.

Deficient blood: see Blood deficiency.

Deficient heat: see *Yin*-deficiency.

Deficient *qi*: see *Qi*-deficiency.

Deficient *yang*: see *Yang*-deficiency.

Deficient *yin*: see *Yin*-deficiency.

Diuretic: Diuretic substances eliminate excess fluids. As understood by Traditional Chinese Medicine, diuretics also enhance fluid metabolism by increasing the body's absorption of fluids into the cells and deep tissues.

Dry, dryness: This state is characterized by dehydration, and is accompanied by the following symptoms: extreme thirst; dry skin, hair, mouth, lips, nose, and throat; dry coughing; and constipation.

Essence: Essence is a highly refined fluid substance; it is the basis of reproduction, development, growth, sexual power, conception, pregnancy, and bodily decay.

Excess: Excess is a condition in which too much of a particular substance (*yin*, *yang*, heat, cold, or fluids) accumulates within the body.

Excess cold: Excess cold is a condition in which the body holds surplus coldness. For a more complete definition of cold, see Cold, coldness, and cold signs, on page 182.

Excess heat: This is a condition in which the body holds surplus heat. For a more complete definition of heat, see Heat, hot, and heat signs below.

Excess yang: see Excess heat, above.

Excess yin: Excess *yin* is an imbalance in which the body holds an overabundance of fluids. Symptoms of this condition include edema, excessive fluid retention, lethargy, a plump or swollen appearance, and overall signs of dampness. Individuals with excess *yin* may move slowly, but they generally have adequate energy.

External, exterior: These terms indicate that the location of an illness is on the surface of the body. External or exterior conditions include colds, flu, fevers, skin eruptions, sore throats, and headaches.

False yang: See *Yin*-deficiency.

Fluids: This term encompasses all fluids in the body, including blood, lymph, intracellular fluids, and cerebrospinal fluids.

Heat, hot, heat signs: This condition consists of hypermetabolism, and is generally accompanied by the following symptoms: fever with slight chills; restlessness; constipation; thirst; aversion to heat and desire for cold; burning digestion; infections; inflammations; dryness; a reddened face; sweating; strong appetite; hemorrhaging; bloody vomit, urine, stools, nose, or mucus; emission of strong odors; sticky or thick, yellow bodily excretions; irritability; scant, dark-yellow urination; swollen, red, and painful eyes or gums; red skin eruptions; and hyperconditions, such as hypertension.

Internal, interior: These terms indicate that the location of an illness is inside the body. Generally, these conditions affect *qi*, blood, fluids, and internal organs.

Jing: see Essence.

Meridians: Meridians are the pathways along which *qi* circulates; they allow *qi* to supply energy and nourishment to the organs and the surface of the body.

Moves blood: see Regulates blood below.

Nervine: Nervine treatments strengthen the nerves; they help heal nervousness, anxiety, insomnia, emotional instability, pain, cramps, spasms, tremors, stress, muscle tension, and epilepsy.

Organs: Traditional Chinese Medicine's (TCM) definition of organs differs from the definition given by Western medicine. In TCM, organs have energetic (rather than physical) functions; they are understood as dynamic, interrelated processes that occur throughout the body. *Yin* organs include the heart, lungs, kidneys, spleen, and liver. *Yang* organs include the small intestine, large intestine, urinary bladder, stomach, and gallbladder.

Qi: *Qi* is energy or life force. It circulates throughout, protects, holds, transforms, and warms the body.

Qi-deficiency: This condition consists of a lack of *qi* or energy. It is generally characterized by the following symptoms: low vitality; lethargy; weakness; shortness of breath; slow metabolism; frequent onset of colds and flu, followed by slow recovery; a low, soft voice; spontaneous sweating; frequent urination; and palpitations.

Regulates blood: This term applies to treatments that smooth the flow of blood in the body. Symptoms indicating the need for blood regulation include bleeding; hemorrhaging; excessive menstruation; localized, stabbing pain; abdominal masses; ulcers; abscesses; and painful menstruation.

Regulates energy: This term applies to treatments that smooth the flow of *qi* in the body. Symptoms indicating the need for energy regulation include dull, aching pain; abdominal distension and pain; belching; gas; acid regurgitation; nausea; vomiting; a stifling sensation in the chest; side pain; loss of appetite; depression; hernial pain; irregular menstruation; swollen, tender breasts; and wheezing.

Sedative: Sedative treatments calm the mind and Spirit. They are used to treat insomnia, anxiety, nervousness, irritability, fright, and hysteria.

Seven Emotions: The Seven Emotions are major contributors to illness. They include sadness, fright, fear, grief, anger, joy (overexcitability), and melancholy.

Shen: *Shen* encompasses an individual's overall Spirit and mental faculties. Qualities of *Shen* include enthusiasm for life; charisma; and the capacity to behave appropriately, respond, speak coherently, think clearly, form ideas, and live a life of joy and spiritual fulfillment.

Spirit: see *Shen*, above.

Stomach heat: This is a condition in which the stomach holds surplus heat. Symptoms of this condition include bad breath, bleeding and swelling of the gums, mouth ulcers, frontal headaches, a burning sensation in the stomach, and extreme thirst.

TCM: This is an abbreviation for Traditional Chinese Medicine.

Tonification, tonify: These terms apply to treatments that nourish, strengthen, build, and improve *qi*, blood, *yin*, *yang*, or Essence.

Wind: Pathogenic wind causes movement or obstruction within the body. Its symptoms include spasms; twitching; dizziness; muscle rigidity; deviations of the eye and mouth, as seen in Bell's palsy; stiff neck and shoulders; tremors; convulsions; vertigo; and sudden onset of colds, chills, fever, stuffy nose, and headache.

Yang: *Yang* defines the body's capacity to generate and maintain warmth and circulation.

Yang deficiency: This is a condition of coldness, caused by the absence of *yang*. Symptoms of *yang* deficiency include lethargy; coldness; edema; poor digestion, accompanied by undigested food in the stools; lower-back pain accompanied by sensations of coldness; constipation caused by weak peristaltic motion; and lack of libido.

Yin: *Yin* encompasses the body's substance, including blood and other fluids in the body. It nurtures and moistens the organs and tissues.

Yin-deficiency: This is a condition in which cooling, moistening fluids (*yin*) are lacking, and bodily heat appears greater than it is. *Yin* deficiency results in emaciation and weakness characterized by heat symptoms; as such, it is called false heat or deficient heat. Symptoms of this condition include night sweats; insomnia; a burning sensation in the palms of hands, soles of feet, and chest; malar flush; afternoon fever; nervous exhaustion; dry throat; dry eyes; blurred vision; dizziness; and nervous tension.

Zang Fu: *Zang fu* is TCM's theoretical explanation of the organs; hollow organs (*fu*) store blood, *qi*, and fluids, and solid organs (*zang*) transform blood, *qi*, and fluids.

Recommended Reading and Sources

Books

Chinese Herbal-Medicine Guides

The following list of materials is not an herbal bibliography, since there is a vast number of valuable books on the topic of Chinese herbology. However, the titles listed below will be of particular use to beginning Chinese-herbal-medicine students. For a more complete bibliography, refer to my book *The Herbs of Life* (The Crossing Press, 1992).

Beinfield, Harriet, and Korngold, Efrem. *Between Heaven and Earth*. New York: Ballantine Books, 1991. This work provides a thorough study of the Five Elements, and details specific herbal formulas and cooking recipes.

Bensky, Dan, and Gamble, Andrew. *Chinese Herbal Medicine: Materia Medica*. Seattle, WA: Eastland Press, 1986. An extensive herbal pharmacopoeia, this reference guide discusses traditional Chinese herbal categories and hundreds of commonly used Chinese herbs.

Connelly, Diane. *Traditional Acupuncture: The Law of the Five Elements*. Maryland: Center for Traditional Acupuncture, 1979. This book offers an in-depth description of the theory behind the fascinating Chinese Five Elements system.

Dharmananda, S. *Your Nature, Your Health*. Portland, OR: Institute for Traditional Medicine and Preventive Health, 1986. *Your Nature, Your Health* contains constitutional diagnoses based on the Five Phases, and includes many Chinese herbs and formulas.

Fratkin, Jake. *Practical Guide to Chinese Patent Formulas.* Portland, OR: Institute for Traditional Medicine, 1986. This book lists 200 patent formulas and their indications.

Hong-Yen, Hsu. *How to Treat Yourself With Chinese Herbs.* Los Angeles: Oriental Healing Arts Institute, 1980. This is a useful introductory guide to the use of Chinese herbs.

Kaptchuk, Ted. *The Web That Has No Weaver.* New York: St. Martin's Press, 1983. This is an excellent beginning guide to Traditional Chinese Medicine.

Lust, John, and Tierra, Michael. *The Natural Remedy Bible.* New York, NY: Pocket Books, 1990. *The Natural Remedy Bible* details natural, herbal remedies for common ailments.

Ni, Maoshing. *Chinese Herbology Made Easy.* Santa Monica, CA: Seven Star Communications, 1986. This herbal guide outlines and compares the specific qualities of many Chinese herbs, in all the herbal categories.

Reid, Daniel. *A Handbook of Chinese Healing Herbs.* Boston: Shambhala, 1995. This handbook gives basic descriptions of over 100 herbs and many herbal formulas.

Tang, Stephen and Palmer, Martin. *Chinese Herbal Prescriptions.* London: Rider and Company, 1986. This book offers good, basic information on Chinese herbs, and includes several cooking recipes.

Teeguarden, Ron. *Chinese Tonic Herbs.* New York: Japan Publications, 1984. *Chinese Tonic Herbs* looks in-depth at most major Chinese tonic herbs; it also provides photographs and prescriptions.

Tierra, Lesley. *The Herbs of Life.* Freedom, CA: The Crossing Press, 1992. A thorough beginners' herbal on Western and Chinese herbs based on the foundations of Traditional Chinese Medicine. Includes specific therapies, remedies, preparations, and food energetics.

Tierra, Michael. *Planetary Herbology*. Santa Fe, NM: Lotus Press, 1988. This extensive herbal guide categorizes herbs from around the world, according to the principles of Traditional Chinese Medicine. It also contains specific remedies for many ailments.

Tierra, Michael. *The Way of Herbs*. New York: Pocket Books, 1980. A great beginners' herbal guide, *The Way of Herbs* categorizes Western herbs according to the principles of Traditional Chinese Medicine. It also contains treatments for specific ailments.

Chinese Dietary Guides

Flaws, Bob. *The Book of Jook*. Boulder, CO: Blue Poppy Press, 1995. This offers an excellent discussion of congees and includes many specific recipes.

Flaws, Bob, and Wolfe, Honora. *Prince Wen Hui's Cook*. Boulder, CO: Blue Poppy Press. This book outlines the principles of dietary therapy, and discusses the use of foods and some herbs in many traditional herb/food recipes.

Jilin, Liu, and Peck, Gordon (editors). *Chinese Dietary Therapy*. Livingstone, NY: Churchill, 1995. *Chinese Dietary Therapy* provides an in-depth look at diet, foods and their therapeutic uses, and recipes (using herbs and foods) for common ailments.

Lu, Henry. *Chinese System of Food Cures*. New York: Sterling Publishing Co., Inc., 1986. *Chinese System of Food Cures* discusses the use of food and herbs to prevent and remedy disease.

Lu, Henry. *Chinese Foods for Longevity*. New York: Sterling Publishing Co., Inc., 1990. This book includes traditional Chinese recipes (using foods and herbs) that promote health and longevity.

Ni, Maoshing, and McNease, Cathy. *Tao of Nutrition*. Santa Monica, CA: Seven Star Communications Group, Inc., 1987. This useful book discusses the energetics of food, and includes remedies for specific diseases.

Educational Resources

"East West Herb Course," taught by Michael Tierra, with Lesley Tierra
Post Office Box 712
Santa Cruz, CA 95061
Phone: (408) 336-5010 or 1 (800) 717-5010
Fax: (408) 336-5010

Three comprehensive, beginning home-study courses in Chinese and Western herbalism are available by correspondence and taught by professionals: Introduction to East West Herbalism, The Home Study Course in Herbal Medicine, or the comprehensive Professional Herbalist Course.

The Introduction to East West Herbalism course is especially designed for the beginning herbal student. The Home Study Course in Herbal Medicine is suitable for beginning students interested in herbal medicine; individuals studying the theoretical basis of the principles of Oriental Medicine and food therapy; and people who sell, grow, or manufacture herbal or health products. The Professional Herbalist Course is directed towards herbal professionals or individuals seeking in-depth herbal knowledge and understanding of the practice of Planetary Herbology. The advanced course synthesizes the first two courses. It will enable you to practice as a competent herbal consultant.

For more information write to the address above.

National Herbal Organization

American Herbalists Guild
Box 746555
Arvada, CO 80006
Phone: (303) 423-8800

The American Herbalists Guild is a professional body of herbalists dedicated to promoting and maintaining criteria for the professional, American practice of herbalism. The Guild also offers student memberships. This organization encompasses herbalists in all aspects of practice, including Chinese, Western, naturopathic, folk, and Native American methodologies. The American Herbalists Guild holds annual meetings in different parts of the country, and publishes a beautiful quarterly herbal magazine called *The Herbalist*.

Weights and Measures

English Measures
a few grains = less than 1/8 teaspoon
60 drops = one teaspoon
one teaspoon = one-third tablespoon
one tablespoon = three teaspoons
two tablespoons = 1 fluid ounce
four tablespoons = one-quarter cup
16 tablespoons = one cup or 8 ounces

Metric Equivalents
one teaspoon = 5 milliliters
one tablespoon = 15 milliliters
one pint = .528 liters
one quart = 1.056 liters
one grain = approximately .65 milligrams
one ounce = approximately 28 grams
one pound = approximately 454 grams
one teaspoon of cornstarch = 3 grams

Index 1: Chinese Patent Medicines

Index 2: Chinese Herbs by Common Name

Common Name	Latin Name	Mandarin-Chinese Name
acanthopanax	*Acanthopanax gracilistylus*	*Wu Jia Pi*
achyranthes	*Achyranthes bidentata*	*Niu Xi*
aconite	*Aconitum carmichaeli*	*Fu Zi*
agastache	*Agastache rugosa*	*Huo Xiang*
alismatis	*Alisma plantago-aquatica*	*Ze Xie*
alpinia	*Alpinia oxyphylla*	*Yi Zhi Ren*
American ginseng	*Panax quinquefolium*	*Xi Yang Shen*
anemarrhena	*Anemarrhena asphodeloides*	*Zhi Mu*
angelica	*Angelica dahurica*	*Bai Zhi*
apricot seed	*Prunus armeniaca*	*Xing Ren*
areca	*Areca catechu*	*Bing Lang*
asparagus	*Asparagus cochinchinensis*	*Tian Men Dong*
astragalus	*Astragalus membranaceus*	*Huang Qi*
atractylodis	*Atractylodes macrocephala*	*Bai Zhu*
biota	*Biota orientalis*	*Bai Zi Ren*
black pepper	*Piper nigrum*	*Hu Jiao*
bupleurum	*Bupleurum chinesis,* *B. scorponeraefolium*	*Chai Hu*
burdock	*Arctium lappa*	*Niu Bang Zi*
cardamom	*Amomum villosum*	*Sha Ren*
carthamus	*Carthamus tinctorius*	*Hong Hua*
chaenomeles	*Chaenomeles lagenaria*	*Mu Gua*
Chinese wild yam	*Dioscorea opposita*	*Shan Yao*
chrysanthemum	*Chrysanthemum morifolium*	*Ju Hua*
cimicifuga	*Cimicifuga foetida*	*Sheng Ma*
cinnamon bark	*Cinnamomum cassiae*	*Rou Gui*
cinnamon twig	*Cinnamomum cassiae*	*Gui Zhi*
cistanches	*Cistanche deserticola*	*Rou Cong Rong*
citrus (see mandarin orange, on page 197.)		
citrus, green	*Citrus reticulata*	*Qing Pi*

clematis	Clematis chinensis	Wei Ling Xian
codonopsis	Codonopsis pilosula	Dang Shen
coix	Coix lachryma jobi	Yi Yi Ren
coltsfoot	Tussilago farfara	Kuan Dong Hua
coptis	Coptis chinensis	Huang Lian
cornsilk	Zea mays	Yu Mi Xu
cornus	Cornus officinalis	Shan Zhu Yu
corydalis	Corydalis yanhusuo	Yan Hu Suo
curcuma, rhizome	Curcuma longa	Jiang Huang
curcuma, tuber	Curcurma longa	Yu Jin
cuscuta	Cuscuta chinensis	Tu Si Zi
cyperus	Cyperus rotundus	Xiang Fu
dandelion	Taraxacum mongolicum	Pu Gong Ying
Dang Gui	Angelica sinensis	Dang Gui
dendrobium	Dendrobium nobile	Shi Hu
dianthus	Dianthus superbus, D. Chinensis	Qu Mai
dipsacus	Dipsacus asper	Xu Duan
eclipta	Eclipta prostrata	Han Lian Cao
ephedra	Ephedra spp.	Ma Huang
epimedium	Epimedium grandiflorum	Yin Yang Huo
eucommia	Eucommia ulmoides	Du Zhong
fennel	Foeniculum vulgare	Xiao Hui Xiang
forsythia	Forsythia suspensa	Lian Qiao
fritillary	Fritillaria thunbergii	Zhe Bei Mu
gambir	Uncaria rhynochophylla	Gou Teng
gardenia	Gardenia jasminoides	Zhi Zi
garlic	Allium sativum	Da Suan
gastrodia	Gastrodia elata	Tian Ma
gentian	Gentiana spp.	Long Dan Cao
ginger, dried	Zingiber officinale	Gan Jiang
ginger, fresh	Zingiber officinale	Shen Jiang
ginger, wild	Asarum sieboldii	Xi Xin
ginseng	Panax ginseng	Ren Shen
ginseng, American (see American ginseng on page 195.)		
gypsum	Calcium sulfate	Shi Gao
hawthorn, berry	Crataegus spp.	Shan Zha
He Shou Wu	Polygonum multiflorum	He Shou Wu

hoelen	Poria cocos	Fu Ling
honeysuckle	Lonicera japonica	Jin Yin Hua
houttuynia	Houttuynia cordata	Yu Xing Cao
isatis	Isatis tinctoria	Ban Lan Gen
jujube dates	Ziziphus jujuba	Da Zao
leaven, medicated	Massa fermentata	Shen Qu
licorice	Glycyrrhiza uralensis	Gan Cao
ligusticum	Ligusticum wallichii	Chuan Xiong
ligustrum	Ligustrum lucidum	Nu Zhen Zi
lily bulb	Lillium brownii	Bai He
lindera	Lindera strychnifolia	Wu Yao
longan berries	Euphoria longan	Long Yan Rou
loquat	Eriobotrya japonica	Pi Pa Ye
lotus, seed	Nelumbo nucifera	Lian Zi
lycii berries	Lycium barbarum	Gou Qi Zi
magnolia, bark	Magnolia officinalis	Hou Po
magnolia, flowers	Magnolia liliflora	Xin Yi Hua
mandarin orange	Citrus reticulata	Chen Pi
mint	Mentha haplocalyx	Bo He
	M. arvensis	
morinda	Morinda officinalis	Ba Ji Tian
morus	Morus alba	Sang Bai Pi
motherwort	Leonurus herophyllus	Yi Mu Cao
mouton	Paeonia suffructicosa	Mu Dan Pi
myrrh	Commiphora myrrha	Mo Yao
notopterygium	Notopterygium incisum	Qiang Huo
ophiopogon	Ophiopogon japonicus	Mai Men Dong
orzya	Orzya sativa	Gu Ya
oyster shell	Ostrea gigas	Mu Li
peony, red	Paeonia lactiflora	Chi Shao
peony, white	Paeonia lactiflora	Bai Shao
perilla	Perilla frutescens	Zi Su Ye
persica	Prunus persica	Tao Ren
phellodendron	Phellodendron amurense	Huang Bai
pinellia	Pinellia ternata	Ban Xia
platycodon	Platycodon grandiflorum	Jie Geng
polygala	Polygala tenufolia	Yuan Zhi
polygonati	Polygonatum sibiricum	Huang Jing

polyporus	*Polyporus umbellatus*	*Zhu Ling*
pseudoginseng	*Panax notoginseng, or*	*San Qi*
(*Tien Qi ginseng*)	*P. pseudoginseng*	
psoralea	*Psoralea corylifolia*	*Bu Gu Zhi*
pueraria	*Pueraria spp.*	*Ge Gen*
radish	*Raphanus sativus*	*Lai Fu Zi*
rehmannia, cooked	*Rehmannia glutinosa*	*Shu Di Huang*
reishi (ganoderma)	*Ganoderma spp.,*	*Ling Zhi*
	especially *lucidum*	
rhubarb	*Rheum palmatum*	*Da Huang*
salvia	*Salvia miltiorrhiza*	*Dan Shen*
saussurea	*Aucklandia lappa*	*Mu Xiang*
scallion	*Allium pstulosum*	*Cong Bai*
schisandra	*Schisandra chinensis*	*Wu Wei Zi*
schizonepeta	*Schizonepeta tenuifolia*	*Jing Jie*
scute	*Scutellaria baicalensis*	*Huang Qin*
siler	*Ledebouriella divaricata*	*Fang Feng*
stephania	*Stephania tetrandra*	*Han Fang Ji*
tribulus	*Tribulus terrestris*	*Bai Ji Li*
trichosanthes	*Trichosanthes kirilowii*	*Tian Hua Feng*
wormwood	*Artemesia annua*	*Qing Hao*
zanthoxylum	*Zanthoxylum bungeanum*	*Chuan Jiao*
zizyphus	*Zizyphus spinosa*	*Suan Zao Ren*

Index3: Chinese Herbs by Latin Name

Latin Name	Common Name	Mandarin Chinese Name
Acanthopanax gracilistylus	acanthopanax	Wu Jia Pi
Achyranthes bidentata	achyranthes	Niu Xi
Aconitum carmichaeli	aconite	Fu Zi
Agastache rugosa	agastache	Huo Xiang
Alisma plantago-aquatica	alismatis	Ze Xie
Allium pstulosum	scallion	Cong Bai
Allium sativum	garlic	Da Suan
Alpinia oxyphylla	alpinia	Yi Zhi Ren
Amomum villosum	cardamom	Sha Ren
Anemarrhena asphodeloides	anemarrhena	Zhi Mu
Angelica dahurica	angelica	Bai Zhi
Angelica sinensis	dang gui	Dang Gui
Arctium lappa	burdock	Niu Bang Zi
Areca catechu	areca	Bing Lang
Artemisia annua	wormwood	Qing Hao
Asarum sieboldii	wild ginger	Xi Xin
Asparagus cochinchinensis	asparagus	Tian Men Dong
Astragalus membranaceus	astragalus	Huang Qi
Atractylodes macrocephala	atractylodis	Bai Zhu
Aucklandia lappa	saussurea	Mu Xiang
Biota orientalis	biota	Bai Zi Ren
Bupleurum chinesis, B. scorponeraefolium	bupleurum	Chai Hu
Calcium sulfate	gypsum	Shi Gao
Carthamus tinctorius	carthamus	Hong Hua
Chaenomeles lagenaria	chaenomeles	Mu Gua
Chrysanthemum morifolium	chrysanthemum	Ju Hua
Cimicifuga foetida	cimicifuga	Sheng Ma
Cinnamomum cassiae	cinnamon twig	Gui Zhi

Cinnamomum cassiae	cinnamon bark	*Rou Gui*
Cistanche deserticola	cistanches	*Rou Cong Rong*
Citrus reticulata	citrus, green	*Qing Pi*
Citrus reticulata	mandarin orange	*Chen Pi*
Clematis chinensis	clematis	*Wei Ling Xian*
Codonopsis pilosula	codonopsis	*Dang Shen*
Coix lachryma jobi	coix	*Yi Yi Ren*
Commiphora myrrha	myrrh	*Mo Yao*
Coptis chinensis	coptis	*Huang Lian*
Cornus officinalis	cornus	*Shan Zhu Yu*
Corydalis yanhusuo	corydalis	*Yan Hu Suo*
Crataegus spp.	hawthorn, berry	*Shan Zha*
Curcuma longa	curcuma, tuber	*Yu Jin*
Curcuma longa	curcuma, rhizome	*Jiang Huang*
Cuscuta chinensis	cuscuta	*Tu Si Zi*
Cyperus rotundus	cyperus	*Xiang Fu*
Dendrobium nobile	dendrobium	*Shi Hu*
Dianthus superbus,	dianthus	*Qu Mai*
D. chinensis		
Dioscorea opposita	Chinese wild yam	*Shan Yao*
Dipsacus asper	dipsacus	*Xu Duan*
Eclipta prostrata	eclipta	*Han Lian Cao*
Ephedra spp.	ephedra	*Ma Huang*
Epimedium grandiflorum	epimedium	*Yin Yang Huo*
Eriobotrya japonica	loquat	*Pi Pa Ye*
Eucommia ulmoides	eucommia	*Du Zhong*
Euphoria longan	longan berries	*Long Yan Rou*
Foeniculum vulgare	fennel	*Xiao Hui Xiang*
Forsythia suspensa	forsythia	*Lian Qiao*
Fritillaria thunbergii	fritillary	*Zhe Bei Mu*
Ganoderma spp.,	reishi	*Ling Zhi*
especially *lucidum*		
Gardenia jasminoides	gardenia	*Zhi Zi*
Gastrodia elata	gastrodia	*Tian Ma*
Gentiana spp.	gentian	*Long Dan Cao*
Glycyrrhiza uralensis	licorice	*Gan Cao*

Houttuynia cordata	houttuynia	*Yu Xing Cao*
Isatis tinctoria	isatis	*Ban Lan Gen*
Ledebouriella divaricata	siler	*Fang Feng*
Leonurus heterophyllus	motherwort	*Yi Mu Cao*
Ligusticum wallichii	ligusticum	*Chuan Xiong*
Ligustrum lucidum	ligustrum	*Nu Zhen Zi*
Lilium brownii	lily bulb	*Bai He*
Lindera strychnifolia	lindera	*Wu Yao*
Lonicera japonica	honeysuckle	*Jin Yin Hua*
Lycium barbarum	lycii berries	*Gou Qi Zi*
Magnolia liliflora	magnolia, flowers	*Xin Yi Hua*
Magnolia officinalis	magnolia, bark	*Hou Po*
Massa fermentata	leaven, medicated	*Shen Qu*
Mentha haplocalyx,	mint	*Bo He*
M. arvensis*		
Morinda officinalis	morinda	*Ba Ji Tian*
Morus alba	morus	*Sang Bai Pi*
Nelumbo nucifera	lotus, seed	*Lian Zi*
Notopterygium incisum	notopterygium	*Qiang Huo*
Ophiopogon japonicus	ophiopogon	*Mai Men Dong*
Orzya sativa	orzya	*Gu Ya*
Ostrea gigas	oyster shell	*Mu Li*
Paeonia lactiflora	peony, white	*Bai Shao*
Paeonia lactiflora	peony, red	*Chi Shao*
Paeonia suffruticosa	mouton	*Mu Dan Pi*
Panax ginseng	ginseng	*Ren Shen*
Panax notoginseng, or	pseudoginseng	*San Qi*
P. pseudoginseng*	(*Tien Qi* ginseng)	
Panax quinquefolium	American ginseng	*Xi Yang Shen*
Perilla frutescens	perilla	*Zi Su Ye*
Phellodendron amurense	phellodendron	*Huang Bai*
Pinellia ternata	pinellia	*Ban Xia*
Piper nigrum	black pepper	*Hu Jiao*
Platycodon grandiflorum	platycodon	*Jie Geng*
Polygala tenufolia	polygala	*Yuan Zhi*
Polygonatum sibiricum	polygonati	*Huang Jing*

Polygonum multiflorum	he shou wu	*He Shou Wu*
Polyporus umbellatus	polyporus	*Zhu Ling*
Poria cocos	hoelen	*Fu Ling*
Prunus armeniaca	apricot seed	*Xing Ren*
Prunus persica	persica	*Tao Ren*
Psoralea corylifolia	psoralea	*Bu Gu Zhi*
Pueraria spp.	pueraria	*Ge Gen*
Raphanus sativus	radish	*Lai Fu Zi*
Rehmannia glutinosa	rehmannia, cooked	*Shu Di Huang*
Rheum palmatum	rhubarb	*Da Huang*
Salvia miltiorrhiza	salvia	*Dan Shen*
Schisandra chinensis	schisandra	*Wu Wei Zi*
Schizonepeta tenuifolia	schizonepeta	*Jing Jie*
Scutellaria baicalensis	scute	*Huang Qin*
Stephania tetrandra	stephania	*Han Fang Ji*
Taraxacum mongolicum	dandelion	*Pu Gong Ying*
Tribulus terrestris	tribulus	*Bai Ji Li*
Trichosanthes kirilowii	trichosanthes	*Tian Hua Fen*
Tussilago farfara	coltsfoot	*Kuan Dong Hua*
Uncaria rhynchophylla	gambir	*Gou Teng*
Zanthoxylum bungeanum	zanthoxylum	*Chuan Jiao*
Zea mays	cornsilk	*Yu Mi Xu*
Zingiber officinale	ginger, dried	*Gan Jiang*
Zingiber officinale	ginger, fresh	*Sheng Jiang*
Ziziphus jujuba	jujube dates	*Da Zao*
Zizyphus spinosa	zizyphus	*Suan Zao Ren*

Index 4: Chinese Herbs by Mandarin Chinese (Pinyin) Name

Mandarin Chinese Name	Common Name	Latin Name
Ba Ji Tian	morinda	Morinda officinalis
Bai He	lily bulb	Lilium brownii
Bai Ji Li	tribulus	Tribulus terrestris
Bai Shao	peony, white	Paeonia lactiflora
Bai Zhi	angelica	Angelica dahurica
Bai Zhu	atractylodis	Atractylodes macrocephala
Bai Zi Ren	biota	Biota orientalis
Ban Lan Gen	isatis	Isatis tinctoria
Ban Xia	pinellia	Pinellia ternata
Bing Lang	areca	Areca catechu
Bo He	mint	Mentha haplocalyx, M. arvensis
Bu Gu Zhi	psoralea	Psoralea corylifolia
Chai Hu	bupleurum	Bupleurum chinesis, B. scorponeraefolium
Chen Pi	mandarin orange	Citrus reticulata
Chi Shao	peony, red	Paeonia lactiflora
Chuan Jiao	zanthoxylum	Zanthoxylum bungeanum
Chuan Xiong	ligusticum	Ligusticum wallichii
Cong Bai	scallion	Allium pstulosum
Da Huang	rhubarb	Rheum palmatum
Da Suan	garlic	Allium sativum
Da Zao	jujube dates	Ziziphus jujuba
Dan Shen	salvia	Salvia miltiorrhiza
Dang Gui	dang gui	Angelica sinensis
Dang Shen	codonopsis	Codonopsis pilosula
Du Zhong	eucommia	Eucommia ulmoides
Fang Feng	siler	Ledebouriella divaricata
Fu Ling	hoelen	Poria cocos

Fu Zi	aconite	Aconitum carmichaeli
Gan Cao	licorice	Glycyrrhiza uralensis
Gan Jiang	ginger, dried	Zingiber officinale
Ge Gen	pueraria	Pueraria spp.
Gou Qi Zi	lycii berries	Lycium barbarum
Gou Teng	gambir	Uncaria rhynchophylla
Gu Ya	orzya	Orzya sativa
Gui Zhi	cinnamon twig	Cinnamomum cassiae
Han Fang Ji	stephania	Stephania tetrandra
Han Lian Cao	eclipta	Eclipta prostrata
He Shou Wu	he shou wu	Polygonum multiflorum
Hong Hua	carthamus	Carthamus tinctorius
Hou Po	magnolia, bark	Magnolia officinalis
Hu Jiao	black pepper	Piper nigrum
Huang Bai	phellodendron	Phellodendron amurense
Huang Jing	polygonati	Polygonatum sibiricum
Huang Lian	coptis	Coptis chinensis
Huang Qi	astragalus	Astragalus membranaceus
Huang Qin	scute	Scutellaria baicalensis
Huo Xiang	agastache	Agastache rugosa
Jiang Huang	curcuma, rhizome	Cucuma longa
Jie Geng	platycodon	Platycodon grandiflorum
Jin Yin Hua	honeysuckle	Lonicera japonica
Jing Jie	schizonepeta	Schizonepeta tenuifolia
Ju Hua	chrysanthemum	Chrysanthemum morifolium
Kuan Dong Hua	coltsfoot	Tussilago farfara
Lai Fu Zi	radish	Raphanus sativus
Lian Qiao	forsythia	Forsythia suspensa
Lian Zi	lotus, seed	Nelumbo nucifera
Ling Zhi	reishi (ganoderma)	Ganoderma spp., especially lucidum
Long Dan Cao	gentian	Gentiana spp.
Long Yan Rou	longan berries	Euphoria longan
Ma Huang	ephedra	Ephedra spp.
Mai Men Dong	ophiopogon	Ophiopogon japonicus

Mo Yao	myrrh	Commiphora myrrha
Mu Dan Pi	mouton	Paeonia suffruticosa
Mu Gua	chaenomeles	Chaenomeles lagenaria
Mu Li	oyster shell	Ostrea gigas
Mu Xiang	saussurea	Aucklandia lappa
Niu Bang Zi	burdock	Arctium lappa
Niu Xi	achyranthes	Achyranthes bidentata
Nu Zhen Zi	ligustrum	Ligustrum lucidum
Pi Pa Ye	loquat	Eriobotrya japonica
Pu Gong Ying	dandelion	Taraxacum mongolicum
Qiang Huo	notopterygium	Notopterygium incisum
Qing Hao	wormwood	Artemesia annua
Qing Pi	citrus, green	Citrus reticulata
Qu Mai	dianthus	Dianthus Superbus, D. chinensis
Ren Shen	ginseng	Panax ginseng
Rou Cong Rong	cistanches	Cistanche deserticola
Rou Gui	cinnamon bark	Cinnamomum cassiae
San Qi	pseudoginseng (Tien Qi ginseng)	Panax notoginseng, or P. pseudoginseng
Sang Bai Pi	morus	Morus alba
Sha Ren	cardamom	Amomum villosum
Shan Yao	Chinese wild yam	Dioscorea opposita
Shan Zha	hawthorn, berry	Crataegus spp.
Shan Zhu Yu	cornus	Cornus officinalis
Sheng Jiang	ginger, fresh	Zingiber officinale
Shen Qu	leaven, medicated	Massa fermentata
Sheng Ma	cimicifuga	Cimicifuga foetida
Shi Gao	gypsum	Calcium sulfate
Shi Hu	dendrobium	Dendrobium nobile
Shu Di Huang	rehmannia, cooked	Rehmannia glutinosa
Suan Zao Ren	zizyphus	Zizyphus spinosa
Tao Ren	persica	Prunus persica
Tian Hua Fen	trichosanthes	Trichosanthes kirilowii
Tian Ma	gastrodia	Gastrodia elata
Tian Men Dong	asparagus	Asparagus cochinchinensis

Tu Si Zi	cuscuta	*Cuscuta chinensis*
Wei Ling Xian	clematis	*Clematis chinensis*
Wu Jia Pi	acanthopanax	*Acanthopanax gracilistylus*
Wu Wei Zi	schisandra	*Schisandra chinensis*
Wu Yao	lindera	*Lindera strychnifolia*
Xi Xin	wild ginger	*Asarum sieboldii*
Xi Yang Shen	American ginseng	*Panax quinquefolium*
Xiang Fu	cyperus	*Cyperus rotundus*
Xiao Hui Xiang	fennel	*Foeniculum vulgare*
Xin Yi Hua	magnolia, flowers	*Magnolia liliflora*
Xing Ren	apricot seed	*Prunus armeniaca*
Xu Duan	dipsacus	*Dipsacus asper*
Yan Hu Suo	corydalis	*Corydalis yanhusuo*
Yi Mu Cao	motherwort	*Leonurus heterophyllus*
Yi Yi Ren	coix	*Coix lachryma jobi*
Yi Zhi Ren	alpinia	*Alpinia oxyphylla*
Yin Yang Huo	epimedium	*Epimedium grandiflorum*
Yu Jin	curcuma, tuber	*Curcuma longa*
Yu Mi Xu	cornsilk	*Zea mays*
Yu Xing Cao	houttuynia	*Houttuynia cordata*
Yuan Zhi	polygala	*Polygala tenufolia*
Ze Xie	alismatis	*Alisma plantago-aquatica*
Zhe Bei Mu	fritillary	*Fritillaria thunbergii*
Zhi Mu	anemarrhena	*Anemarrhena asphodeloides*
Zhi Zi	gardenia	*Gardenia jasminoides*
Zhu Ling	polyporus	*Polyporus umbellatus*
Zi Su Ye	perilla	*Perilla frutescens*

OTHER RELATED NATURAL HEALTH BOOKS

An Astrological Herbal for Women
By Elisabeth Brooke
An extensive guide to the use of herbs in healing the mind, body, and spirit, organized by planetary influence. Brooke describes the mythological history and astrological significance of 38 common herbs, as well as their physical, emotional and ritual uses.
$12.95 • Paper • 0-89594-740-4

Good Food: The Complete Guide to Eating Well
By Margaret Wittenburg
An indispensable, comprehensive food guide and nutritional resource. "Good Food makes good sense for anyone interested in shopping smart for eating well." -Bob Arnot, author of *Turning Back the Clock*
$18.95 • Paper • 0-89594-746-3

The Herbal Menopause Book
By Amanda McQuade Crawford, M.N.I.M.H.
Offers a wealth of natural self-care therapies for women during the "change".
$16.95 • Paper • 0-89594-799-4

The Herbs of Life: Health & Healing Using Western & Chinese Techniques
By Leslie Tierra
"Directions are especially clear with a good bibliography and resource guide. A nicely done addition to the popular literature." —*Library Journal*
$16.95 • Paper • 0-89594-498-7

The Information Sourcebook of Herbal Medicine
By David Hoffman, M.N.I.M.H.
This reference offers a bibliography of herbalism and herbal pharmacology, a glossary of herbal and medical terms, a guide to computer databases for the herbalist, and Medline citations for commonly used medicinal herbs.
$40.00 • Cloth • 0-89594-671-8